GOOD HEALTH
AND
COMMON SENSE

By the same author:

ARTHRITIS AND COMMON SENSE
COMMON COLD AND COMMON SENSE
HEALTHY HAIR AND COMMON SENSE
DRY SKIN AND COMMON SENSE

GOOD HEALTH

AND

COMMON SENSE

BY

Dale Alexander

WITKOWER PRESS, INC.

WEST HARTFORD, CONN.

Library of Congress Catalog Card Number: 60-13133

ISBN #911638-03-2

Printed in the United States of America

2nd printing May 1974
3rd printing August 1974
4th printing November 1974
5th printing January 1977
6th printing July 1977
7th printing March 1978

To you, the reader . . .

because your very interest in this book proves that you
care about your health.

You have chosen this volume because you are
seeking to protect your body from illness . . . and because you are searching for knowledge and peace of
mind.

This book is dedicated to you . . . because you are
willing to use common sense to achieve a better way
of life.

Contents

GOOD HEALTH
AND
COMMON SENSE

Chapter I

The Key to Better Health

You and I have the same goal . . . the same interest . . . as we start this book together. We are seeking the answer to one question: "How can I live a longer, healthier and happier life?"

In these pages it is my assignment to point the way, giving you the latest facts and new ideas. Here is a "plan of action" to combat illness. No matter what your age, you can learn how to improve your future by reading these chapters. They are designed to help you feel better, longer.

The problems of advancing age—most of the ailments that afflict man—can in my opinion all be traced to one common cause: improper nutrition. And the best method to counterattack against disease is through the food we eat.

You are the most important factor affecting your health and you are the one to whom health is the most important thing in the world. Your family, those who love and need you, may give you every care and devotion, but no one can be with you every moment of the day, no one can know every feeling, desire or appetite that you have. Doctors can help enormously and, at times, they are the only ones who can help, but you

3

cannot be their only concern; they cannot know everything about you; they cannot be with you all the time.

So you are the only one who can hold the key to
your good health. The name of that key is COMMON
SENSE and the purpose of this book is to show you how
to use it to achieve a longer, healthier, happier life for
yourself.

There are a number of elements that determine the
condition of your body, such as your constitution, your
physical activity, your mental attitudes; but obviously
the most important matter is what goes into your body,
what you eat, drink and inhale. Not only what you eat
and drink is crucial but also when and how. It has been
said that you are what you eat. Of course, this is not entirely true, but there is a good deal of truth in that
statement.

I am not a doctor, psychiatrist, physical-culture expert or reducing specialist. I am not going to prescribe
medicine, delve deeply into mental health, recommend
exercises, weight or figure improvement. Common sense
can be brought to bear on all these matters, but far and
away the most important area for your use of common
sense is your diet—what, when and how you eat and
drink. And that's what I am going to tell you about in
this book.

I believe that the best way to prevent and fight
most of the ailments that afflict mankind is through
proper diet and nutrition.

With proper diet and nutrition you will feel better, you will have good body tone, you will have pep and you will avoid being constantly tired and listless.

MY APPROACH TO THE BETTER UNDERSTANDING OF HEALTH

My approach to the study of human nutrition differs from any other in the world. This is not in any way to take away from the vast amount of work which has been done in this field and each day brings new knowledge. But it is my belief that the relationship of oil-free liquids to the oil-bearing foods in the diet makes the difference between health and poor health.

As far as I know, I am alone in insisting that only whole milk or soup be the choice of liquid with all meals.

The one thing that seems to me to make the essential difference between good health and something less than good health, is the improper use of water in relationship to the food that we eat. I maintain that the best way for you to help water to contribute to your health is by drinking it at the proper times before and after eating, not during meals.

My approach to the study of nutrition also includes emphasis on the difference between the two kinds of sweets and the two kinds of starches in the carbohydrate family. One type helps the body and the other leads to illness. Also, there will be an effort made to alert readers to the two kinds of oils in our foods, good and bad. Your health may depend on this kind of knowledge.

In addition, my dietary system makes use of cod-liver oil consumed in a special way.

I firmly believe that diet and nutrition can solve many of the mysteries which still puzzle medical science. In this book I'll tell you why. Most important. before I make any suggestions in the field of diet, I will detail the efforts, fact-finding and study that led me to write this book.

How My Interest in Health Matters Began

My story really begins 25 years ago, when I was a schoolboy in Connecticut. My interest in the subject of better health was sparked by a situation in my own family. My mother was a victim of arthritis, and I decided to study the disease. Seeking a method to relieve her pains and arthritic problems, I started my research and first concentrated on this illness: I traveled to libraries throughout Connecticut, reading everything I could find on the topic of arthritis. I consulted medical textbooks, health magazines, technical publications—always searching for a clue that could help all arthritics.

Shortly before World War II—before I entered the armed forces—I had determined that proper diet was the answer. Mother's arthritic condition responded favorably when she followed my dietary rules. Throughout my service in the Air Force, I continued searching for an answer to this crippling illness. Upon returning to civilian life, I settled in New York City to study further and to see my dietary plan tested among other arthritics. A doctor in New York began using my nutritional approach among his patients, with success.

The next step was to place my theories about arthritis in written form. I hoped to distribute copies to doctors, hospitals and to some people with arthritis so that they could try this plan of diet. In order to have my ideas set in type, we needed money for a printer. My wife and I took all our savings (even cashed in our war bonds) to pay the printing bill.

All we had was a manuscript, which I had titled *Arthritis and Common Sense*. Our only purpose was to circulate some copies, to have my menus used by actual arthritics. We were determined to prove that my dietary regimen was an effective method of fighting illness.

I sincerely felt that if enough people were helped by my arthritic diet, then medical science would recognize the results. Perhaps then I could work with doctors and scientists to conduct extensive tests, tests to show that better nutrition is the answer to major diseases.

What actually happened is still a surprising and dramatic story. It is a truly American success story. I never set out to "write a book," never had the slightest intention of becoming an "author." Yet, after *Arthritis and Common Sense* * was placed between book covers, it soared to number one on the best-seller lists across the nation. More than 700,000 copies are already in circulation in this country alone.

There were hundreds of radio and television appearances, plus a series of lectures from coast to coast. And I did all this for just one reason. It gave me a chance to reach millions of people. My message was finally being heard; I could now convince a vast audience that diet is the key to better health!

Television made it possible for me to contact a tremendous number of viewers. But, actually, it was my lecture tour that was most important.

I still remember my first speaking engagement in Los Angeles and I shall always be grateful to the men

* Published by Witkower Press, Hartford, Connecticut.

and women who came to hear me that day. They were arthritics, and believed in what I had to sȃy. They tried my dietary plan and followed my suggestions on nutrition.

Soon results began to show. Many experienced relief, improvement, and they told others about my recommended diet. By word of mouth—people telling other people—the good news was spread across the nation. Requests came in for me to speak and I traveled to more than 100 different cities to answer questions about arthritis.

After each lecture, members of the audience would meet with me to describe their experiences and their arthritic problems. From them I learned new facts and ways to improve my dietary program. During these travels, in city after city, I also talked with doctors and visited clinics—constantly searching for more information.

Later in this book I will go into a more detailed discussion about *Arthritis and Common Sense* and controversies surrounding it. I mentioned it here only to show how I got started on my study of diet. My conclusions were that if diet was a key element in arthritis it could very well be a key element in many other ailments. So I broadened my study and research into other areas of health.

The Search for the Common Sense Key to Better Health

Stated simply, my approach to problems of health is to collect facts, examine the research of medical authorities through the years and then apply common sense.

Most great discoveries—in every field of science—were made in the same way: by studying proven facts, by collecting evidence already in existence and by being able to see a common link in all this information.

The discovery of vitamins is an excellent example. Casimir Funk, a biochemist, believed that natural foods contained elements which belonged to the group of chemical substances called amines. Funk set forth his "Vitamine Theory" back in 1912. Actually, he made no new discoveries of his own. Instead, he studied existing facts and was wise enough to recognize a connecting link which made all the previous research make sense.

It had already been proven experimentally that natural foods contain substances that are vital to life. Scientists were already aware that these substances were different from fats, protein, carbohydrates, mineral salts and water.

These facts were known because of experiments performed by Lunin with live mice in 1888. He took all of the food elements known at that time and fed these in purified forms to the mice; they could not survive on this "artificial" diet. However, when the mice were given a "natural" diet of bread and milk, they flourished. Therefore, the "natural" foods must contain something besides the known ingredients.

Earlier research had also suggested that beriberi, scurvy and possibly rickets seemed to be caused by the lack of something in the diet. At this point in history Casimir Funk published his theory that there were four different "vitamines" in foods and that the lack of these "vitamines" would cause four different diseases: beriberi, scurvy, pellagra and rickets.

This was the start. Other vitamins were discovered later, but these original observations by Funk formed the basis for future research. Incidentally, like anyone exploring new areas of thought, Funk made some errors. Not all of his views were completely correct. For instance, Funk believed that all vitamins were amines, a class of chemical compounds. (That's why he named them "vitamines"—amines which are vital to life.) Today, this is known to be untrue. But it does not alter the importance of his original theory, which embraced the idea that many diseases stem from a common cause, many disorders have a common denominator.

Benjamin Franklin expressed this idea in its simplest terms.

For the want of a nail the shoe was lost.
For the want of a shoe the horse was lost.
For the want of a horse the rider was lost.

For want of a rider the battle was lost.
For the want of a battle the kingdom was lost.
And all for the want of a horseshoe nail.

There are many "nails" in the human system, elements or ingredients that we get in our food that are as important to our health as that horseshoe nail was to that kingdom. When that battle was lost it was probably difficult to diagnose the cause—the want of a horseshoe nail. Likewise it may seem hard to believe that some tiny element in a diet—or lacking from a diet—is the cause of a serious disease. But you will see that is so in many—and possibly most—cases.

The human body is a complex of chemical elements. Predominantly these are carbon, hydrogen, oxygen and nitrogen. But there are many other elements which are required, even though each may contribute only a tiny percentage. Perhaps this factor is easier to understand if we compare it to the relationship of iron and steel. Steel is well over 90 per cent iron. But a small percentage of carbon will convert the iron to steel of one type, a small percentage of tungsten will convert the iron to steel of a much tougher type, and so on.

This human-body complex of chemical elements is generally in balance, but it is a precarious balance. As a practical matter it is impossible to keep the composition exactly the same. Every breath we take, every move we make, every moment of passing time affects the balance, however slightly. The human body is constantly working, using up and disposing of some of its material every instant in its life.

To replace the used-up, disposed-of elements, we eat and drink and thereby try to replenish the supply of chemicals that constitute our body. <u>And this is the core of the whole matter of health.</u> If the supply of food and drink is sufficient—containing enough of all required ingredients in correct proportion—the body will flourish. If it is insufficient, if it lacks some of the needed elements or if the proportions are wrong, the precarious balance will tip, the complex will get out of order, the body will weaken and deteriorate. You will be sick.

Properly, when all the elements you take into your body are assimilated in an orderly way, the whole machinery of your system works smoothly and you are in good health. Improperly, when the supply is wrong, there are failures in the series of chemical combinations, one miscombination causes another and you don't feel good, you are vulnerable and finally you will have a disease.

Critics will claim that I am ignoring bacteria and viruses. My answer is simple. I maintain that a human body will not be so susceptible to bacteria or viruses if the person has been eating the right foods to build up advance resistance.

Infectious diseases—from bacteria and viruses—could not gain a foothold unless the body were already vulnerable, weakened by a type of "malnutrition." If you have been eating the wrong foods, depriving your body of a truly healthy diet, infection strikes.

From the day we are born, proper nutrition controls our growth and our degree of health.

As I have said, this book is concerned with the key factor of health, the matter of diet—the supply of materials to your body. There are other factors, of course, such as the viruses and bacteria just mentioned, and the air we inhale, which may be country-pure or sodden with smog or filled with gasoline fumes or saturated with tobacco smoke. But I maintain that these are secondary factors and there are a host of them. The primary foundation of good health is proper diet, the primary cause of bad health is improper diet.

Proper Foods and Correct Eating Habits

Which foods are best to prevent or alleviate illness? What dietary mistakes should we avoid to gain better health?

The answers to these two questions will form the theme of this book. Read on, and you will discover complete chapters devoted to both of these subjects. A list of recommended foods and menus will be found in Chapter XX. Balanced diets are discussed in detail in Chapter IV.

But right here at the start I would like to emphasize one key fact about natural foods. I strongly advocate that we should eat our foods in a form as close as possible to their natural and raw state. I am very alarmed about the trend toward using more and more highly processed foods.

According to my observations, eating habits have already reached a point where a majority of the people in the United States now live on a diet which consists of 20 to 60 per cent processed foods. These foods did contain natural elements. But during processing these elements are often rearranged into an unnatural form; many food values are lost or lessened in effectiveness.

You read on wrappers or boxes, "vitamins A, B, C, etc., added." Most of the natural values of the food have been destroyed, so synthetic vitamins are substituted. Is this done to pacify the consumer or to ease the conscience of the manufacturer?

I am going to classify foods in two different ways: (1) natural or raw, (2) processed or cooked. As I said I am convinced that natural and raw are best. It is true that usually the only foods generally edible in their natural, raw state are fruits, vegetables, certain shellfish, milk directly from the cow, eggs and nuts in the shell and a few other things like honey, herbs, spices. Even raw meat has been processed to some extent, and every grain that reaches our kitchens has been processed to some extent. Cooking is a process too. Whether you boil, broil or fry the food, you affect its composition to some degree. Most moderately processed foods are good, and I accept them and use many of them as you will see in my menus. It is the highly processed foods that I try to exclude and I think you should avoid in your diet.

Many "modern-day" diseases were unknown centuries ago. The types of illness that afflicted mankind 5,000 years ago were far different from the ailments of today.

> **Early men, and primitive people today, were dependent on natural foods. They did not eat any processed foodstuffs, which lack certain needed elements and contain other needed elements but in strange combinations that are unfamiliar to the body and possibly unworkable. Examples are whipped butter, hydrogenated peanut butter, processed cheeses. When we began to consume vast quantities of highly refined foods we became victims of a flood of "new" diseases.**

It is my belief that the present widespread incidence of nervous disorders, heart trouble, arthritis, etc. has been caused in part by our increased use of processed food and the consequent lack of certain needed elements which were eliminated during the processing.

To obtain the proper natural foods for your daily diet requires increasingly more attention on your part because there are so many unnatural foods now on the market. You must be constantly on guard. To add a sufficient number of "health foods" to your normal menu is not a chore. You will suffer little inconvenience, and your meals can be as tasty as ever. To learn how, consult Chapter XX.

Balance the Liquids and Solids in Your Diet

There have been many discussions and many books written that supposedly reveal a "balanced diet." Nutrition experts have described how to maintain a balance between meats and vegetables, how to balance minerals and vitamins. But little attention has been paid to oils in the diet. Fats are mentioned but oils are treated as part of fats. Actually, oils are a crucial factor in diet. Oil-bearing foods and liquids play an important part in diet, as do also oil-free liquids. Milk and most soups are oil-bearing. Water, coffee, tea are oil-free liquids which can be wrong for you at times.

Can liquids help the digestion of a meal and facilitate the distribution of the food elements through the system? Or do they dilute or lessen the food value of solids? We all know that water is essential to the human body. But is there a wrong time to drink water? Does it complicate or spoil the process of digestion? Because these are important questions, I have covered thoroughly the relationship between liquids and solids in our daily diet. Likewise, other key factors are fully discussed and the answers given in later chapters. Right now, to make the whole subject clearer I have compiled a list of ten items you should know and understand, a chart that can be your guide to a healthier, happier life.

TEN IMPORTANT FACTORS THAT DETERMINE
OUR HEALTH

1. Correct diet.
   Proper utilization of foods in order to get their values.
2. "Natural" foods (to strengthen our daily diet).
   Dangers of devitalized foods.
3. The correct preparation of foods.
   Retaining of food values in storing and cooking.
4. The relationship of liquids to solids.
   Consumption of oil-free liquids and solids so that they do not conflict during digestion.
5. Water intake.
   Indiscriminate use of drinking water can be harmful.
6. The proper food temperatures during meals.
   Avoid congealing your foods.
7. Proper circulation.
   Avoid "blood-sludging" in your system.
8. Emotional and nervous tension.
   Modify stress and strain through proper nutrition.
9. Heredity.
   Imitating family eating habits can contribute to the "inherited tendency" of disease.
10. Virus and bacteriological infections.
    Increase resistance through diet correction.

You will note that all the key factors in the chart center around food, water and nutrition. These subjects are so important that you need far more information than just a list of "recommended" foods.

In the chapters ahead we must consider food selection, preparation, digestion. And we shall also consider "right" versus "wrong" oils in the average diet.

Then, in addition, I shall give you a specific list of

a complete set of day-by-day menus. They are outlined for you in Chapter XX.

Upon reading them, you will find that many of these menus could be classified as part of an "oil-bearing diet." The emphasis is to provide the necessary oils in your system, for use by your body. Proper oil supply or "lubrication" of your bodily joints can be an important safeguard for your general health. The oils do not literally lubricate the joints, but derivatives from oils do nourish them and provide elements that appear to be essential to the good condition of the joints and joint linings.

A Clinical Evaluation

The value of a diet bearing proper oils has been proven. Not long ago, a series of scientific tests was made to determine whether my recommended diet would produce good results. A medical center in New England conducted a clinical evaluation of my dietary regimen.

This project at the clinic began in order to prove my findings in regard to arthritis. Nine years ago, when my book on arthritis was first published, I advanced the theory that proper diet could alleviate arthritic pains and problems. In that book I listed foods and oil-bearing diets which were followed by thousands of readers with excellent results.

But the medical profession could not recognize this plan for arthritis unless or until it could be substantiated through a clinical evaluation.

So that's exactly what was done. Tests were made on a group of actual patients, unselected cases of arthritis coming through that medical center in New England. They were started on my dietary regimen. The group included patients with osteo, rheumatoid and mixed types of arthritis. There were cases covering all stages of the disease—early, moderate and severe.

For a period of nearly six months each patient followed the recommended dietary plan and was periodically examined at the clinic. Tests included X rays, blood chemistry, sedimentation rates and all the recognized procedures of a formal clinical study. The progress of each patient was carefully recorded, and these results were published in the *Journal of the National Medical Association* (July, 1959).

After the patients had faithfully followed our plan, their health changed dramatically. Here are some actual excerpts from the final report of the clinical evaluation.

"Ninety-two per cent of the patients responded to the dietary regimen with improvement within periods of two to twenty weeks."

". . . marked reduction of pain, and general improvement in well-being of the majority of the patients."

". . . diminished tissue swelling, improved range of motion and mobility, less fatigue, better complexion, frontal [forehead] signs of luster, skin and scalp improvement, re-established levels of earwax, stronger nails and much more alertness."

Yes, we now have positive proof that proper diet plays a role in the fight against arthritis. When I learned the official results of this clinical evaluation, it was one of the greatest moments of my life. To know that your findings are correct, your theories proven, is the finest possible reward. The years spent in research, the hard work, all seemed worthwhile.

I tell the story of this clinical test for a very specific reason: during this same study at the clinic we discovered many new facts about diet. It became evident that my dietary plan would also be beneficial to combat other diseases. My original diet had been designed for arthritics. But now it was possible to make modifications and changes, to apply a similar theory to help victims of other ailments.

As I explored each different illness, one fact became clear: I was not alone in my belief that proper nutrition is the key, the answer to a wide variety of health problems. Scores of doctors and recognized medical scientists are also convinced of this.

Throughout this book, I shall list by name many of the prominent physicians who are actually conducting experiments and research in the field of nutrition.

You now have a preview of the subject matter which you will find in these pages. This will be a logical account, a case built on facts. The decision will then be yours. "Eat, Drink and Be Healthy!"

Chapter II

Danger Signs . . . And How To Read Them

The mirror of your future health is the way you look and feel today. The mirror on your wall can reveal whether you are really well . . . or whether you are eating your way into illness and infirmity.

It is definitely possible to predict certain ailments by self-examination in your own mirror at home. Preliminary symptoms can be recognized easily, if you know what to look for and how to interpret what you see.

Before I list the "danger signs"—so you can check your own reflection—let me make one point very clear. I am not proposing that you rely solely on self-diagnosis. If you feel ill, go to your doctor for a complete physical and laboratory test. But I do maintain that you can anticipate many illnesses—and perhaps prevent them— by taking a close look at yourself, now.

Face up to the fact that your complexion, your eyes, ears, hair, etc., all reflect your inner health. They can serve as a barometer and warn you of health complications ahead.

Complexion is a helpful guide. I often wonder why most people are only interested in the complexion of children. When they see a baby or growing youngster, they almost always comment: "Look at those rosy cheeks! This is certainly a healthy child." What about adults? Why don't we pay more attention to cheek-coloring in older people?

I'm certainly in favor of a woman using rouge and make-up. But she's only fooling herself if beneath it all she is a pale, undernourished candidate for illness. Men are guilty of the same complacency with their barber-shop "sun tans."

Conversely, an excessive redness of cheeks in adults may be a symptom of trouble, probably high blood pressure.

Let Your Mirror Speak

Tomorrow morning—before applying that lipstick or shaving off that beard—take a good, close look. Start by examining your EYES, and ask yourself these questions:

> Do your eyes appear dull, have they lost their brightness and luster?
> As there any encrustations in the corners?
> Are the eyelids red-rimmed?
> Is there puffiness at the lower rims of your eyes?
> Do you suffer from burning eyes and dimness of vision?
> Are there fatty deposits (patches or tiny mounds of cholesterol) in eyelids and around the eyes?

If you answered "Yes" to any of the above questions, your diet may be at fault, and it's time to take corrective measures.

Now hear this . . . examine your EARS. Check these warning signals:

Are your ears particularly pale, lacking in color?
Is there a scaliness in or around the canals of your ears?
Do you experience "buzzing" and ringing noises?
Is there dryness, a lack of earwax?

Too little earwax is a definite symptom of an oil deficiency. Improper eating habits—and the wrong foods with insufficient or incorrect oils—are causing your blood stream to fail to deliver specific dietary oils where they are needed in your body. One place you can easily detect body-oil shortage is in your ears, where earwax can serve as an indicator. No wax will develop if no oil or not enough oil is reaching your ears (and therefore not reaching other parts of your body). In the absence of the needed oils, the tiny ear ossicles begin to harden. The auditory system starts to break down. Slowly, through the years, real damage is caused to the inner ear. *Would you rather wear a hearing aid in later life, or correct your diet now?*

The symptoms we have just described—in regard to eyes and ears—can be summarized in two words: dietary deficiencies. You are missing important food elements and you should realign your meals.

The results of faulty nutrition can also be observed if your mirror shows the following problems:

Is your hair too dry, lifeless-looking?
Are you troubled with dandruff?
Are you becoming bald, or is your hair turning prematurely gray?
Is your diet causing your hair to be excessively oily?
Do you have dental worries, a rapid rate of decay?

Does the tip of your tongue seem too red? (If it is a darker red than the rest of your tongue, you may be on your way to a vitamin deficiency.)

Is your complexion marked by acne, eczema, black-heads or other unsightly blemishes?

Does the skin of your cheeks, nose or forehead show enlarged pores?

If you are a woman, do you tend to have excessive hair growth on your face?

All of these minor mysteries of health are telltale signs that illnesses can soon develop. There are exceptions to the rule, certainly—conditions caused by infection, congenital defects, or injuries. But in the majority of cases, I do maintain that all these afflictions are basically caused by faulty nutrition. Beyond the age of thirty, as we grow older, more and more signs appear.

Many people, when they suspect that their diet is at fault, will rush right out and buy some vitamin pills. Unfortunately, it takes more than just vitamins, minerals or a bottle of capsules. The best solution is to think in terms of "dryness" . . . realize the fact that your body is "drying out." Take steps which will add lubrication to your system!

Certain foods contain dietary oils that have oil-soluble vitamins and specific fatty acids. These oils will restore the luster to your skin, will lubricate a dry scalp, will replenish earwax, will aid other body functions, ease body activities. Most of the symptoms described in this chapter will respond to a series of oil-bearing meals. Follow the menus listed in Chapter XX.

I repeat: a common cause of illness is a general

"dryness" throughout the human body. However, the answer is not entirely the <u>selection</u> of "oily" foods. After you have chosen the items for a menu, you must understand <u>how</u> and <u>when</u> to eat the various parts of a meal. Otherwise, the full value of the "oils" will be lost.

It is still necessary to observe a <u>balanced diet.</u>

There is a right way—and a wrong way—to balance your daily menus. This subject is so vital, I shall devote an entire chapter to the matter. But first I want to outline the course which food follows through your body. It's important to understand how your body handles the food and liquid you consume.

Chapter III

The Body's Feed Line

Among all the remarkable structures of the human body the digestive system may well be the most intriguing. There is still much to be learned about the details of its mechanism, but enough is known to evoke the awe of anyone who investigates it. But it is very important to remember that there is still much to be learned, that many mysteries remain in the amazing complex of the digestive process.

The physical plant of the digestive system consists of a long tube with an opening at each end. There is considerable variation in the diameter of the tube; it follows no straight line but rather weaves back and forth, turning on itself many times. The inner surface is covered with projections, convolutions and ridges. The tube extends from the upper opening, the mouth, by which food enters it, to the anus, from which waste products leave it. (Perspiration and urination also serve to dispose of waste.)

The Digestive Process

The process of digestion can be described in very general terms as follows: The food is before you. You

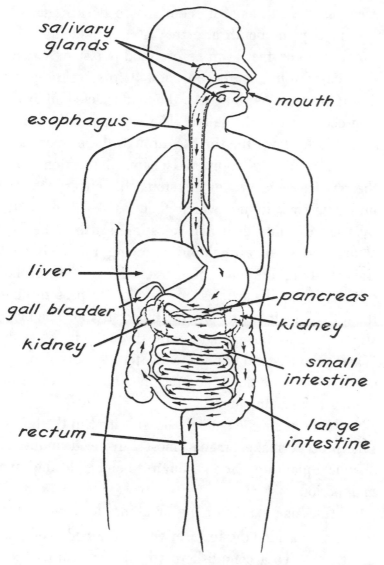

salivary
glands

mouth

esophagus

liver

gall bladder

kidney

pancreas

kidney

small
intestine

large
intestine

rectum

THE BODY'S FEED LINE

see it, smell it, think of it. Your senses alert the salivary glands in your mouth and they start producing juices containing enzymes even before food is tasted. When it does enter your mouth you chew it to start the grinding-up process. As you chew, the food is acted on by certain chemicals in the saliva. The wet, partially ground mass moves down the throat, through the esophagus to the stomach. Here additional chemical reactions, plus the physical churning of the stomach, convert the food into a viscous liquid, which then passes through the pyloric valve into the small intestine. Further chemical changes keep digesting and reducing the food as it travels along the intestinal tract. Here it is broken down into small particles fine enough to pass through the wall of the intestine into the blood stream. The blood stream carries the food to cells throughout the body. Waste products and undigested materials move from the small intestine to the large intestine and on through the rectum to be eliminated.

It seems simple enough, doesn't it? But the how of this process makes man's most advanced industrial chemical plant appear as though it belongs to the caveman period.

Take one example: the breaking down of protein into amino acids (the form in which the body cells can use them). To accomplish this in the laboratory, man must bring the protein to the temperature of a blast furnace, add concentrated acid weighing ten times the weight of the material and boil the mixture for twenty hours. The digestive system accomplishes this same feat in about three hours, using a much weaker acid at body temperature—98.6°. To illustrate further the efficiency of enzymes (the chemicals produced by the body to assist digestion) it has been proven that one ounce of the proper enzyme from a hog's stomach will digest 50,000 ounces of boiled egg white in two hours.*

Enzymes Are Necessary

Knowledge about enzymes has increased at a rapid pace in recent years, but biochemists realize that a vast field remains to be explored. It is currently believed that every living cell uses enzymes to effect chemical change. Since there are so many diversified cells creating so many different kinds of reactions, it seems probable that the number of enzymes produced in the body far exceeds any previous notion about them. For our purposes, however, we will discuss only the most important: those whose functions relate directly to the digestive process.

In the saliva of the mouth ptyalin is found. This enzyme acts on starches so that on reaching the stomach they are broken down into simpler forms.

It is estimated that the stomach contains 35,000,-000 glands which secrete hydrochloric acid, mucus, pepsin, rennin, lipase and at least one hormone, gastrin. The pepsin and the acid begin the breakdown of the

* E. Borek, *Man, the Chemical Machine* (New York: Columbia University Press, 1952).

complex protein molecules. The mucus lines the stomach walls, protecting them from damage by the acid. Rennin coagulates milk protein, lipase starts the reaction on fats and the hormone controls the speed of the chemical action.

While all this activity is taking place, the muscular stomach walls are pulsating, churning and crushing the food until it becomes semiliquid. The liquid stream then passes into the small intestine, where it is subjected to pancreatic juice. This is formed by the pancreas and contains the enzymes trypsin, chymotrypsin, amylase and lipase; and intestinal juice containing at least five more enzymes, as well as bile produced by the liver. Here the final breakdown of fats, proteins and starches takes place and the food is able to pass through the intestinal wall by the process of osmosis.

Surrounding the intestinal wall are large numbers of thin-walled blood vessels into which the food stream passes. Now the food is carried by the blood stream to every one of the many billions of cells in the body. Each of the cells uses the food for its special purpose—the building of bone, tissue, fat, nerves, creation of coverings like the nails and hair, conversion into energy, blood cells, enzymes, hormones and innumerable other products necessary to the continued functioning of the incomparably complex human body.

Nature has provided wonderfully for the digestion of the food you take into your body, but you have to provide the food in (a) sufficient supply, (b) digestible form, (c) under suitable conditions. Explained in greater detail:

(a) There must be enough of all the elements needed by the body. Your body can extract the needed elements from food but it cannot manufacture them.

(b) If the food is not in soluble form it will pass through your body unused. Corn on the cob is an example. Each kernel is covered by a sort of natural cellophane. If you do not chew through this covering, your enzymes will not be able to reach the meat of the kernel; and it will pass through your body, completely undigested. There are many other ways in which food you consume may be blocked off entirely or partially from the digestive process. You can help in this respect by chewing your food thoroughly.

(c) You have to be concerned not only with what your food supply must contain but also with what it must not contain. Certainly you won't knowingly consume poisons, but you may unknowingly be consuming them. In many processed foods nowadays there are tiny quantities of chemicals which can in time make trouble for you. Elements that are natural are likely to be compatible with your digestive system. However, there are many excellent natural substances which may prove quite harmful to your digestion if consumed at the wrong time so that they interfere with the digestion of other foods. Obviously anything excessively hot or cold is bad, but there are times, as we'll point out, when even such things as drinking water may be wrong.

Your Health Depends on Which Way Your Dietary Oils Are Absorbed

At this point I want to make it clear that my approach to the matter of diet and digestion is unique. I favor strongly the use of natural organic foods and I oppose strongly the use of processed, denatured foods. But I am not alone in that, and I think that in time all the weight of expert opinion will be on the side of natural foods. However, I am alone, at this writing, in my "oil factor" doctrine. *I believe that the proper use and distribution of oils in the body makes the difference between good health and bad health. And I am convinced . that the liquids you drink (during or near meals) determine whether you will have proper, effective distribution of oils or bad, ineffective and harmful distribution of oils in your body.*

We have just followed in a general way the course of foods through the body. The course of oils is the same as all other foods until the splitting of the components is accomplished in the small intestine. At this point, approximately 70 per cent of the oils passes through the lymph vessels into the bloodstream, and approximately 30 per cent passes through the liver, eventually into the heart and then into the blood stream.

But these percentages are seriously affected by liquids consumed at the time the oils are being digested. Liquids are very helpful in the digestive process. We need them. Liquids like whole milk and soup, which have low surface tension, will not affect the normal course of the oils. But high-surface-tension liquids, like ordinary drinking water, will interfere with the dietary oils. Oils do not mix with water. The water does not absorb the oil particles but rather "surrounds" them, acting to some degree as an envelope or a barrier. It is more difficult for the lymph vessels to absorb the "surrounded" oil particles, and therefore the lymph vessels miss some of the oil they would otherwise accept. The lymph vessels never absorb all the oils in any case. But instead of absorbing 70 per cent, as is normal, they absorb perhaps as little as 50 per cent when the oils are partially "covered" by water.

It is true that the stomach juices and the action of the stomach will reduce the high surface tension of the water, but the tension will still be higher than liquids like soup or milk.

Water has the highest surface tension, but other high-surface-tension liquids, like coffee, tea, etc., will act in the same way, though in lesser degree.

In the case of ice-cold liquids, which shock the stomach and impede its working, the wrong-way percentage is even greater and perhaps only 30 per cent of the oils will reach the system through the lymph vessels. In the meantime, while the oil-supply is deficient, some parts of the body will be starved for oils and will be definitely affected by the lack of their needed elements.

What happens to the diverted oils? They pass into

the liver and cause extra work for that organ, which must break them down, reduce them to fragments. In this process the liver extracts the vitamins and the key ingredients from the oils and retains them, thereby enriching itself, making it healthier and wealthier at the expense of other parts of the body, which become impoverished, frail, weaker, disordered and finally sick. The residue is passed along through the circulatory system, some in readily soluble form, some almost insoluble. When the less soluble oils reach the coronary arteries, they may stick and tend to clog the artery passageway. Some of this oil does reach the needy areas, but since it has lost much of its quality and many of its ingredients it can serve as fuel but cannot be properly effective as a "lubricant."

However, very little attention has been given by nutrition experts and physicians to the digestive system's oil routing. But I am convinced that it is a crucial matter affecting health. At the moment there is no real scientific data on the subject; no clinical tests have been conducted to establish the course of the oil, one way or the other. But for the practical demonstration of my point I have ample evidence.

You Must Learn How To Drink a Glass of Water

For many years, in my book and in my lectures on arthritis, I have been counseling a special water-drinking regimen: no water or other high-surface-tension liquid from fifteen minutes or more before mealtime to at least four hours after a meal. I don't know how many of the more than 700,000 people who bought my book and the millions of people who have heard me in lectures, on television and radio, have followed my water-drinking regimen. But undoubtedly many thousands have done so and many, many have reported to me—"Great improvement"—"Dryness corrected within weeks"—"Quick relief!" These people insist that they have gained great benefit from this regimen. And I am sure no physician can say there is any possible harm in it.

Water is necessary to human life, and your health depends on an adequate supply. Medical science tells us that our bodies require a cubic centimeter of water for every calorie our foods produce. Therefore, if you follow a diet containing 2,100 calories per day, you need approximately 2,100 cubic centimeters of water. This is the equivalent of eight glasses of water!

No one would be foolish enough to recommend that you "drown" yourself by drinking eight glasses of water every day. Many foods contain great quantities of water. Milk, for example, is 87 per cent water. Soup has an even higher percentage. Most fruits, vegetables and meats are actually more than 50 per cent water.

Millions of Americans who are now living normal, healthy lives drink as little as one glass of water daily. Their bodies do not become "dehydrated," nor do they suffer any ill effects.

However, let's never be complacent and look upon

water as a "harmless" liquid. There are some definite dietary dangers involved.

There is no need to "wash down" your food with a glass of water at mealtime. Instead of helping your body, you may be hindering the digestive process, you may be detouring needed food elements, you may be causing extra work for your body, as will be explained later.

Some individuals crave more water than others, at more frequent intervals. It is my belief that a well-balanced body chemistry rarely manifests a great or constant thirst for water. If you are trying to adjust to my dietary plan (or at any time when you are thirsty), you will find that a piece of celery, carrot, cucumber or fresh fruit will usually meet your thirst needs.

Then during the day, if necessary to satisfy thirst, water may be taken approximately four (or more) hours after a meal or other food intake, or about half an hour before a meal.

Most foods have within themselves the necessary amounts and types of water for their own solubility. Drinking water with meals is a false and useless attempt to speed up digestion. Let your food be "broken down" with the aid of protein, fat and carbohydrate digestive enzymes and food-splitting acids. This is a natural function of the body.

The more slowly food is absorbed the more it is exposed to the intestinal flora and the less chance there is of constipation.

I have sometimes been asked why I am so adamant against water, why I issue so many warnings on the subject. Let me clarify my stand by repeating that I am actually in favor of drinking water—but only at certain times of the day. The timing is what counts.

Drink water to your heart's content upon arising, 30 to 60 minutes before breakfast, and again about half an hour before the evening meal. Be guided by the following simple rules:

1. **No water with your meals or midway between meals.**
2. **NO ICED WATER AT ANY TIME.**
3. **Never add water to milk. (Obviously, I do not recommend powdered milk.)**
4. **Never add water to soup to cool it.**
5. **If you must drink coffee (which is water, with high surface tension) do so at least fifteen minutes before breakfast. If you feel that you must have coffee during the day, then drink it black, preferably at least 30 minutes before your noon and/or evening meal and four hours after your previous meal.**
6. **Avoid using flavored, carbonated water, or seltzer. (Social occasions sometimes require that you take a drink. A "straight Scotch" or "Scotch and water" would be better than a "Scotch and soda." Better still, abstain.)**

Readers of my first book have also asked another key question: "What about drinking water when I take pills, tablets, vitamins and other medication?"

The answer is try to take capsules and medication with water early in the morning, upon arising. Another "safe" time is about 30 minutes before the evening meal. If your prescription requires pill-taking more than twice a day, perhaps you can use milk as the accompanying liquid.

Since writing my book on arthritis, which includes an entire chapter on how to drink water, I have learned that in some East European countries there is a taboo against drinking water during meals. This is an ancient tradition that is still observed. Perhaps we can learn something from it.

My simple before-and-after demonstration is not precise scientific proof, but it is clearly convincing: BEFORE abstaining from water in the meal period: dry skin, painful, inflamed joints, poor body tone. AFTER a few weeks or a few months of mealtime abstinence from water: smooth, lustrous skin, well-lubricated, easy-acting joints, good body tone. Obviously the water-timing was the key factor.

In pointing out how water may be bad for you at times, I do not want you to forget how good and necessary water is for you at the right times. In pointing out how good and necessary oils are for your body, I do not want you to forget that there are good and bad oils. In the same way you know that food is good and essential for you, but there are of course good and bad foods. But don't forget that there are now, and increasingly as time goes on, many bad forms of good foods. All these matters, and how to use your common sense in choosing the foods and liquids you consume, will be covered in later chapters.

Chapter IV

Why "Balanced" Diets Often Fail

In recent years there have been dozens of "balanced diets" offered to the American public. Books, magazines, daily newspapers—all have championed some special diet. Millions of words have been published to prove that certain menus contain the proper number of calories, vitamins, etc.

Unfortunately, most of these dietary planners have all made one common mistake: they neglected to mention the three main factors which can "unbalance" any menu ever designed. They spent too much time telling you which foods to select, and they kept giving you elaborate charts on calorie-counting.

Meanwhile, however, many of these health experts forgot to warn you about three important rules. No matter how wisely you choose your foods for any meal, you must also pay attention to these three facts:

1. **The order in which you eat your food.**
2. **The temperature of food when it is served.**
3. **The preparation of food, the method of cooking.**

The "balance" in a balanced diet will definitely disappear unless you follow the proper procedure in these three areas. Your food cannot be digested and assimilated correctly if you ignore any of the three points listed above. You want full assimilation—full value from the food you consume—so you must consider all three.

As you read on, throughout this book you will find complete discussions of all three subjects . . . the recommended order of eating foods, the best temperatures for serving food, the recommended methods of food preparation. But right now let's investigate this key topic of diet assimilation. Let me give you one interesting example.

A Dutch physiologist named Pekelharing conducted an unusual experiment. His work proved how one food element can vitally affect the whole system. He first performed this test way back in the year 1905, but the results are still valid today.

The experiment began with a group of white mice. They were fed a diet containing proteins, carbohydrates, fats and the necessary salts and water. Their "menu" included bread baked with casein, albumin, rice flour, lard and a mixture of all food salts.

The liquid chosen for the white mice to drink was water. WITHIN FOUR WEEKS, ALL THE ANIMALS WERE DEAD.

Simultaneously, another group of white mice was fed the identical diet. But, for a liquid, they were given milk. Four weeks later, all these mice were hale and hearty, in excellent health.

These findings by Pekelharing were also corrob-

orated by Dr. G. Hopkins, a Nobel prize winner. Dr.
Hopkins did research on "synthetic diets," also using
mice, and published his report in 1912. In this experiment, small amounts of milk (2-3 cc.) were added to
meals consisting of synthetic foodstuffs. It made the
difference between life and death.

Modern research continues to show that milk is
helpful as we assimilate our daily diet. One good example could be the Seventh Day Adventists. This reli-
gious group is known to drink more milk—and less
coffee and alcohol—than the average. It is quite possible that this wise course is an important factor in their
general good health.

A survey has been under way for several years
among 60,000 Seventh Day Adventists throughout California. In April of 1958 a report was given to the California Medical Association by Dr. Ernest L. Wynder of
the Sloan-Kettering Institute of Cancer Research in New
York, and Dr. Frank R. Lemon from the College of
Medical Evangelists in Loma Linda, California. Their
hospital records showed 90 per cent less cancer cases
and 40 per cent fewer heart attacks among Adventists
compared to non-Adventists!

The impressive size of this study—among 60,000
persons—makes it a real contribution to science. And,
in view of the results, I consider it a fine testimonial to
the value of milk as a dietary aid.

Drink Milk To Reduce "High Tension"

As I have said, the way to obtain maximum benefit from the food you eat is to select and drink the right liquids at mealtime. Whole milk, for instance, is most helpful—because it has low surface tension and it will assist your body to assimilate other foods.

Milk has oil-soluble vitamins within its liquid state. Without such oil-soluble vitamins, bodily organs lose their power to assimilate the principal parts of food. The secret is to avoid, at mealtime, liquids that have high surface tension. Avoid water, coffee, tea, soft drinks. Rely on whole milk!

This subject—the surface tensions of various liquids—could explain the different degrees of health in your entire family. Suppose the mother, father and the children all eat the same kinds of food every day. Part of the family maintains a good record of health, yet others in the same household have a tendency to develop repeated illnesses. Why?

One reason can be the drinking habits, the choice of beverage with meals. One member of the family eats a sandwich and washes it down with soda pop. Another person at the same table takes two or three cups of coffee during the luncheon. Perhaps someone sips from a glass of ice water throughout the meal. Most probably, only the children use milk as the main beverage.

My point is this: within one family there can be

a wide variety of drinking habits. All members may eat the same solid foods, but they take different liquids, at different temperatures, at different times in relation to the meal. (Even this timing is important—you must know which liquids to drink before your meals and which to drink during the meals, and after you finish eating.)

All these factors can affect the "balance" in an otherwise balanced diet. Is it not reasonable to conclude that different beverages can cause your digestive system to react in different ways? If you have just enjoyed a glass of whole milk—rich in oil-soluble vitamins and food values—what happens to it if you immediately drink a glass of cold water? You have added a liquid with high surface tension, you have forced your body into extra effort to assimilate the beneficial elements of the milk.

In a way, this phase of good nutrition is a war between the liquid and solid portions of your diet. Within the same family, some people win—and some lose. It all depends on daily habits of eating and drinking—and a little will power and some common sense!

Enjoy Your Foods in the Proper Order

There is a science to the order of eating. Certain foods conflict with each other during the process of digestion and assimilation . . . so we must understand when to eat each food during the course of the same meal.

When foods reach the stomach they can react upon one another. In certain cases we may lessen or nullify the food values before they have a chance to be distributed throughout our blood stream.

Many parts of your body require oil-soluble vitamins for specific nourishment. My dietary program—including the menus listed in Chapter XX—is designed to give you the "oils" you need for better health.

When I use the expression "dietary oils," I mean those oils in foods that contain oil-soluble vitamins, the unsaturated fatty acids, organic iodine and other natural factors. The following foods are the most important sources of high-grade nutritional dietary oil:

Cod-liver oil
Whole milk
Butter (unsalted, not whipped)
Natural cheeses
Fish body oils

In contrast, I want you to know that I am opposed to the "inferior food oils," such as those contained in oleomargarine, bacon grease, ice cream, chocolate, foods cooked or heated in vegetable fats, hydrogenated fats, hydrogenated peanut butter, whipped butter, whipped cream cheese and all meat fats, including the hidden fats in sausages and cold cuts.

An excess of wrong oils in the blood stream serves to undermine the balance of health.

The meals I have planned for you are based on

proper lubrication through correct eating habits. I want to make it clear, once again, that I use the term "lubrication" for the purpose of simplicity. The dietary oils do not provide a film to avoid friction, but the properties peculiar to them do provide a unique kind of nourishment to the joints and help them to work better. The result is comparable to that of lubrication.

To protect the oil-bearing food in your diet, remember this famous truth: Oil and water do not mix. I repeat—liquids if taken at the wrong time during a meal, can rob the oils of some of their potential power. Instead of "lubricating" your system, the same oils may end up as "energy." Oil-soluble vitamin A—instead of strengthening your eyes—can become a handicap to your liver or just add to your waistline.

Of all the words in the world of nutrition, there is one which holds the key: assimilation. Everything revolves around this one subject. For example, your ability to assimilate also depends on how your food is prepared. Cooking, baking, broiling, roasting or frying—each method can either add or detract from your health in the long run.

Scrambled eggs give you less nutritional value than the soft-boiled variety. That is because it is much easier for the yolk of a soft-boiled egg to be assimilated and travel through the blood stream to benefit your body.

Meats should never be overcooked. Why destroy or disperse the very vitamins you are cooking? Broil your meats, medium rare.

Vegetables are fine, as long as you avoid excessive cooking that will draw nutritional values out of the vegetables into the water, or into the air. Better still, serve vegetables raw, whenever possible.

Throughout this book you will find many helpful facts about the preparation of food—how to avoid losing your food values, how to preserve proteins, minerals and vitamins. But by now perhaps you have recognized some of the errors you may have made in regard to your own daily diet.

The Answer to Those Dietary "Danger Signs"

In a previous chapter, I asked a number of questions about what you see in your mirror. You were given the "danger signs"—but not the actual cause of each symptom. Now that we know more about balanced diets in general, let me give you some specific answers:

If your eyes appear dull and lack luster, there are three likely reasons: (1) Defective assimilation of your food. (2) Not enough oil-soluble vitamin A. (3) Wrong oils in your diet, which are nullifying the oil-soluble vitamin A.

Encrustations in the corners of your eyes can be a deficiency of unsaturated fatty acids (which are best found in cod-liver oil).

Puffiness and swelling beneath the eyes is often due to improper assimilation. Burning of eyes and dimness of vision probably indicate a deficiency of riboflavin.

Fatty deposits of cholesterol in eyelids and around the eyes can be caused by wrong oils in your diet. You may also have poor fat metabolism, a deficiency of unsaturated fatty acids and defective assimilation.

If your ears seem particularly pale, you should suspect anemia. The liquids and solids in your diet may be "out of balance"—not in their proper relationship.

Scaliness in or around the canals of your ears often indicates a deficiency in the food you eat, a lack of unsaturated fatty acids. If you often hear "buzzing" or ringing noises, chances are that you suffer from an inadequate supply of vitamin-B complex. Too little earwax is due to the defective assimilation of your food. Your diet does not contain the proper "oils," and you may soon become a victim of "blood-sludging." (A detailed description of "sludging" will be found in Chapter VI.)

Hair problems, too, may be directly related to your daily diet. Baldness can result from a lack of "sprouting" foods (foods, like onions, that continue their growth after being taken from the soil and can stimulate the germinating cells of the scalp), vitamin B, sulphur and other minerals. Dandruff can occur when your foods contain too little biotin. You may be eating too many sweets when you really need more vitamin-B complex.

Dry hair which has lost its luster is a sign of poor fat metabolism. You are not gaining enough unsaturated fatty acids, and you need better blood circulation. If your hair and scalp are excessively oily, then you may be eating foods containing the wrong "oils"—and these foods are being improperly assimilated.

Dental troubles (a tendency to cavities) can be traced to a deficiency of fluorine, vitamin D and calcium.

When your tongue becomes red and sore, your diet may be extremely low in niacin. Acne and similar blemishes can occur from eating too much white sugar. This same white sugar—plus too many refined foods—can also cause enlarged pores. Excessive facial hair growth is often due to an imbalance of hormones.

From all these examples—the "danger signs" we have just described—it is easy to see how <u>diet</u> and <u>nutrition</u> affect your entire body. Every area of health is controlled by what you eat!

Most people are vaguely aware that their daily diet may lack certain elements. They suspect that they are not receiving enough "vitamins"—or they worry about "carbohydrates" and "calories."

The people who attend my lectures always ask a great many questions about vitamins. So . . .

Some Answers About Vitamin Pills

Taking a vitamin tablet—to supplement your daily meals—can be a wise move. But be careful, because there are many types of commercially manufactured vitamins. Read the label on the vitamin bottles, and be sure that the capsules are <u>not</u> prepared from coal-tar or aniline chemicals—they lack enzymes and other complementary factors.

Try to be certain that the substances in the vitamin tablets come from natural sources, that they were grown in organically treated soil, free from chemical fertilizers and pesticides. If you obtain your vitamin tablets from health-food stores, which are alert to these factors, you are likely to get the right kind of tablets.

In addition to vitamins, many people take mineral supplements in capsule or liquid form. There is no harm in this. Your body needs many minerals. The most important are calcium, phosphorus, iron, iodine—plus the trace minerals like copper, zinc, etc., which are just as essential. You can get all of these elements, however, from three foods: milk, green vegetables and lean meat.

Proteins and Carbohydrates

The basic fact to remember about proteins is that nearly 50 per cent of your daily diet should consist of protein. The best sources are lean meat, poultry, fish, milk, cheese, eggs and seed cereals.

Throughout this book we will be discussing "fats" and "oils"—their value to your general health. In our enthusiasm for an oil-bearing diet, let's not overlook one other essential factor. Let's mention, now, the role of carbohydrates—the starches and sugars.

Your daily meals must include a generous percentage of high-quality carbohydrates. Unfortunately, the carbohydrates in refined "sweets" (cake, pie, candy) are deficient in value, may be worthless and in some instances can be actually harmful. Once inferior sweets enter the blood stream they "unbalance" the value of the natural sweets. Instead, you should take comb honey, dates and fresh raw fruits as the only kind of sweet in your diet.

Another good source of carbohydrates is whole grain cereal and bread. Ordinary white bread (refined and highly processed) has often lost the beneficial carbohydrates. Again, inferior starches "unbalance" the meal.

Nutrition Expert States His Case

One of the nation's foremost nutritionists—Dr. Clive McCay of Cornell University—has gone on record to predict the future of diet versus disease.

"Dr. McCay believes that heart disease, arthritis, diseases of the bone and teeth, and kidney diseases all will eventually prove vulnerable to the nutritional approach!"

He maintains that many ailments of old age are nutritional ailments due to faulty diet or inadequate utilization of food by the body. "Poor nutrition," he stated, "may be caused by an excess, an imbalance or a dietary deficiency in certain elements." He reported his views before the Gerontological Research Foundation in St. Louis.

This good news—that proper diet may soon offer the answer to crippling illness—was published in the St. Louis *Democrat* (May 25, 1957). Since then, there has been added progress, in another direction. More and more, our nation is being warned about the poisons in our foods.

Chapter V

Enemies of Health

POISONS, NEAR-POISONS, THE DANGERS OF
SMOKING AND DRINKING

My sole object in this book is to tell you what and how to eat and drink so that you can be healthy and happy. And with this, of course, I aim to tell you what not to eat and drink so you won't be ailing, in pain, or sick.

But there are some things you can't or won't do, some evils you can do nothing or little about, some dangers you will choose to risk. Many books have been written about each and every one of these well-recognized evils and dangers. But I will simply flag them and emphasize the need for you to exercise some care and use your common sense in dealing with them.

Poisons

In this day and age there are poisons all around us: in the air we breathe, in the food we eat, in the liquids we drink. I refer not only to atomic fallout but also to the many, many poisons used in this Chemical Age to grow, treat, protect and preserve foods. In the aggregate, these food chemicals constitute a much greater danger than strontium 90.

Our air may also be contaminated with chemical and gasoline fumes, DDT and other insecticide and pesticide sprays. Not only do we inhale this contaminated air but the animals that will provide our food breathe it, are affected by it.

I am not with the calamity-howlers who see the world coming to an end as a result of this, but any intelligent person must recognize it as an evil that requires government attention.

Food producers, from cattle ranchers and poultry breeders to farmers and food-processors, use all sorts of chemical additives to fatten their stock and to stimulate faster growth. They add chemicals to make foods last longer or look better. They add chemicals to enrich, fortify or hydrogenize them. Some of these chemical additives are poisons, but of course the amount of the poison is tiny, a mere trace. Yet in some cases these traces are retained in the body, and trace added to trace can add up to an effective dose. There are federal laws prohibiting or controlling the use of chemicals in foods, but perhaps some revision is needed. The Department of Agriculture is vigilant, though of course not perfect in enforcing and policing these laws. But apart from joining in a campaign for better laws and better enforcement, what can you as an individual do to protect yourself?

Well, the important thing is to be on guard. The

law requires that the ingredients of packaged foods be listed on the label. Read the labels—especially the fine print. Remember that the processor merely has to list the ingredients—he does not have to explain or describe them. When you see any chemicals listed, you are seeing a danger flag. Of course, the amount contained may be harmless. Benzoate of soda is a poison, but 1/10 of 1 per cent is considered a harmless amount, and the Food and Drug Administration permits it. Nevertheless you should realize what you are consuming.

As for unpackaged foods—fruits, vegetables, meats—try to find out as much as you can about them. The simplest thing is to examine them closely. Some fruits and vegetables are covered with a thin film of paraffin to make them look better, last longer. Some oranges, meats and even vegetables are artificially colored. They are not exactly what they seem. By inquiring you can often find out the source of the food—New Jersey eggs, Massachusetts cranberries, Texas tomatoes. This source of information can be helpful if you try to learn which are the good areas for certain foods and which are dubious.

Finally—how did it taste? Any aftereffects? The answers to these questions will help to guide you in your food-shopping.

I don't want to minimize the harm of these trace poisons in your food, but potentially much more harmful are the quasi poisons in processed foods—the nonpoisonous isomeric* elements in processed foods that can result in much more harm to you than actual poisons. These elements are thoroughly discussed.

Smoking and Drinking

People smoke tobacco because it gives them pleasure, relaxes them, gives them the satisfaction of indulging themselves. People drink liquor because they think it stimulates them, enables them to feel at ease, helps them to forget their problems. But they pay for it. Every smoker, every drinker should realize what his indulgences are costing him. Too often the price is excessive.

If these habits are followed with moderation, it is possible to enjoy reasonably good health. But the odds are against it.

A package of cigarettes contains a collection of poisons—carbon monoxide, nicotine, arsenic, hydrocyanic acid, coal tar and ammonia. All these are found in cigarette smoke. When and if you inhale, you make them available to your blood stream. Inhaled smoke has a detrimental effect on your heart. Smoking causes a rise in blood pressure, an increased pulse rate and certain changes in the pattern of an electrocardiogram. In time there are also changes in the circulation. The

* When two or more compounds have the same percentage composition but differ in the relative positions of the atoms and have different properties, they are called isomeric compounds. The natural food element is one that the body is accustomed to; an isomer of it may be strange to the body because of this difference in structure, and therefore may not be so readily assimilated.

arteries narrow and the skin temperature falls. Cigarette-smoking especially leads to constriction of the small blood vessels. Smoking can result in cold hands and legs and can affect your breathing. . . . All this from nicotine.

As for tobacco tar and nicotine causing cancer, conclusive evidence is lacking. Yet tobacco tar is a chemical irritant and nicotine interferes with the oxygen content of the blood. In due time, in my opinion, smoking will prove contributory to cancer if the diet is simultaneously at fault.

Smoking interferes with the appetite. Smokers, on the whole, eat less than nonsmokers. This may seem like a good thing to people who want to keep their weight down, but the chances are that the body or certain elements or areas of the body are being undernourished and eventually trouble will come of it as the effect accumulates.

My advice about smoking is DON'T, but I know many people will go on smoking, even knowing the hazards. To them I say that attention to proper nutrition is all the more important. The right diet may enable you to afford this indulgence that is so costly to your health.

Alcoholic liquor has its uses and values and is often prescribed medically. Many doctors advise their older patients to take a little whiskey or brandy each day as a helpful stimulant for the heart.

The trouble is that too many people drink too

much alcohol; their behavior is influenced to some degree by the alcohol and they may become intoxicated.
Even in moderate amounts, alcohol always has a de-
pressive effect and its action on the higher cerebral
centers can cause a loss of self-control and a weakening
of will power.

The drinker loses his appetite and does not eat
enough; his body is undernourished, starved for proteins, vitamins and minerals. His digestion is thrown off
balance not only by the alcohol but by the ice or the
iciness of most alcoholic drinks. And in the bodily
process of burning up the alcohol as fuel, other vitamins
are drained off. Even after the "influence" or the "in-
toxication" has passed, the body does not work right
because its supply of certain vital elements is insufficient.

The first noxious effects of alcohol are manifested
in the brain. Even the smallest amounts of alcohol have
been shown by careful experiment to reduce the accuracy
of movement requring muscular coordination. The special senses of sight, hearing and touch become less keen.

As the amount of alcohol ingested is increased,
emotional instability and slight motor incoordination
are followed by confusion, staggering gait and slowed
speech. The effect is cumulative and the chronic drinker's
body will be chronically below par.

Long-continued alcoholism may lead to a psychosis,
hallucinations, paranoia accompanied by a state of deterioration from the permanent organic changes in the
brain.

Clearly the wisdom is not to drink alcohol except for medicinal purposes. If at any time you do drink to excess, remember that in your diet you have to repair the damage to your body. You have to replenish by proper nutrition the supplies of needed elements that were depleted by the alcohol.

Excesses

Common sense calls for moderation in all matters of eating and drinking. Most people are aware of the danger of certain excesses—liquor, sweets, coffee, carbonated beverages, etc. But you can also have too much of a good thing like salt, especially if it is refined salt rather than the mineral salts found in natural foods. Keep down your use of pepper, spices and heavily spiced foods and the oil-free beverages you drink to overcome those "tangy aftereffects." Any excess can cause trouble for your body.

Lack of Sleep and Rest

Lack of sleep is of course a real danger to the body. No matter what the other factors are that are causing your sleeplessness, the right diet will help you to sleep better. And perhaps a fundamental cause of your sleeplessness was wrong diet in the first place.

There are many reasons why a person may be restless or nervous, but as in the case of sleep, the right nourishment will ease the situation. And perhaps the wrong nourishment, the lack of certain elements needed by the body was the original cause of the restlessness, or a contributing factor.

Chapter VI

How To Feed Your Heart

The problem of heart disease may soon be materially reduced. This encouraging news is more than just a hopeful prediction. Medical science has already learned the most important facts, and a great campaign against coronary ailments can now begin.

If the scientists and research men will merely follow the evidence which is now before them, then the battle is essentially won. Some experts believe that the cause and control of heart disease are both related to cholesterol. I agree. In fact, I maintain that the control of cholesterol—through diet and proper nutrition—is the basic approach for those seeking a healthy heart.

The importance of cholesterol (pronounced ko-less-turr-all) will be discussed throughout this chapter. So, first, let's understand the word itself. For a definition, we go to *Dorland's Medical Dictionary*. . . .

> CHOLE—combining form denoting
> relationship to bile
> STEROL—stiff, solid

CHOLESTEROL is a fatlike, pearly substance found in all animal fats and oils, in bile, blood, brain tissue, milk, yolk of egg, the medullated sheaths of fibers, the liver, kidneys and adrenal glands.

If a doctor suspects heart disease, it is already accepted procedure to check the patient's blood—determine the level of cholesterol in the blood stream. The body cannot survive without cholesterol. But too much may be harmful.

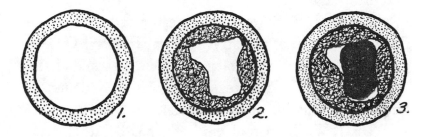

1. Normal artery wall. 2. Fatty deposits begin to collect. 3. Passage is narrowed. Blood supply may be closed off if blood-clot forms.

Many conservative cardiologists regard the presence of excessive amounts of cholesterol in the blood as one of the factors leading to the onset of coronary disease. Therefore, they recommend steps to lower the blood cholesterol level. The trouble alleged to be caused by cholesterol is clogging of the arteries. The thought is that cholesterol particles cling to the interior walls of arteries and thereby tend to close up the passage. The heart must pump harder to get the blood moving through the narrowed arteries and therefore suffers extra strain.

I believe the medical world is on the right track in

following this line of research. Some important contributions have been made to our knowledge in this field. For instance . . .

Dr. E. H. Ahrens, Jr., of the Rockefeller Institute, New York, and his colleagues were among the first to recommend that we should reduce our intake of cholesterol-bearing foods.

Dr. J. M. R. Beveridge, professor and head of the Department of Biochemistry, Medical Faculty, Queens University, Kingston, Ontario, Canada, was one of the first to favor the use of vegetable (corn) oils (unsaturated fatty acids) to reduce cholesterol.

Dr. J. W. Gofman of the Donner Laboratory, University of California at Berkeley, and his associates, demonstrated that blood cholesterol levels could rise on a low fat diet when the carbohydrate portion was increased. Dr. Gofman tells about this in his book, *Dietary Prevention and Treatment of Heart Disease.*

Dr. B. Bronte-Stewart, now of the Oxford University Medical School, has reduced cholesterol by utilizing highly unsaturated vegetable and fish oils.

Dr. O. W. Portman, Harvard University School of Public Health, Boston, Massachusetts, and his co-workers have studied the relationship between cholesterol and a diet high in refined sugar. (Their finding: a diet high in refined sugar increases blood cholesterol levels.)

Dr. L. M. Morrison, medical director of several hospitals in Southern California, has discovered that de-fatted soya-lecithin is highly effective in reducing blood serum cholesterol. He found also that adding brewers' yeast and wheat germ to the diet was effective in the prevention and treatment of heart disease. Soya-lecithin has the ability to keep the blood-stream oils in finer emulsion and thus of greater potential help to the body. It aids in the manufacture of cholinesterase, an enzyme needed for better health.

Research on rats being done by the United States Department of Agriculture at Beltsville, Maryland, has turned up new laboratory clues. It has found that ordinary white sugar may play a role in the body's production of excess cholesterol. Sugar is now on the lengthy list of foods suspected of causing trouble in the heart and arteries.

Said a representative of the research group: "There are five major food categories—fats, carbohydrates, protein, vitamins and minerals. All of them have been under suspicion at one time or another."

I want to point out that there are six, not five, major food categories. Water is the sixth major food category. I wrote to the United States Department of Agriculture about this. The answer to the letter agreed:

Water is often considered a food category, in which case it would be the most essential of all. . . . Water is provided ad libitum in our diet studies using laboratory animals; we have made no studies in which water intake was controlled. We know of no studies testing the effect of meals with and without water on blood serum cholesterol in man. . . .

It is time water and its relationship to the entire meal, as well as to cholesterol, was studied.

The Danger of Wrong Oils

To maintain the proper level of cholesterol within our bodies we must learn to avoid "wrong oils" in our daily diet. Which oils are wrong and which oils are right? What makes an oil bad or good? The best you can do is make a generalization, and this will require some judgment and common sense on your part.

To begin with, oils that turn solid at room temperature are the wrong oils. Meat drippings, if allowed to cool on your plate, turn into fats. These are saturated fats. They are saturated with hydrogen, and they are not good for the body. Why not? Because they are chemically less active and are poorly utilized by the body. You can easily recognize saturated fats; they do not turn rancid easily and do not pick up odors from other foods. They are inactive substances, so to speak.

The human body must use or get rid of the fuel it takes in. Unsaturated oils help the body to get rid of the relatively inactive saturated oils.

Let us return to the meat drippings. The very fats they come from, then, are all saturated. Therefore, any fat in any meat is bad. When you look at a piece of steak, or uncooked hamburger filled with fat, you are looking at fats which are solid at room temperature. If you take these into your body, they will finally be utilized but poorly. And to be utilized, they need help from oils that are chemically active, the unsaturated fats. The reason why unsaturated fats can help alleviate your dietary mistakes is that unsaturated fats either have iodine or can borrow some iodine from your endocrine glands or some reservoir supply. Unsaturated fats are known to be chemically active. They, by a process known as double bond exchange, can "loan" the saturated oils in your system some precious iodine. But this is done at the expense of your metabolism and health. No matter how much your intake of unsaturated fats can help correct the damage of the saturated fats, some internal degeneration develops in the body.

PROTECT YOUR HEART . . . CAREFULLY SELECT YOUR DIETARY OILS *

UNDESIRABLE DIETARY OILS (saturated fats)	GOOD DIETARY OILS (unsaturated fats)	BEST DIETARY OILS (unsaturated fats with higher iodine content)
Meat fat drippings	Corn oil	Cod-liver oil
Chicken fat	Soybean oil	(especially good when
Bacon fat	Sunflower seed oil	of dark color and rich
Sausages, hot dogs, and all cold cuts containing "hidden" fats	Safflower seed oil	in iodine)
	Sesame seed oil	Fish body oil
	Cottonseed oil	Whole milk
All meat fats	Olive oil	Eggs (The yolk is excellent if the egg is soft boiled or poached.)
Chocolate and candy	Unroasted peanut oil	
Whipped butter	Other plant-derived oils (These oils still lack or are deficient in organic iodine.)	
Oleomargarine		
Whipped cream cheese		
Hydrogenated peanut butter		
Potato chips	Creamery butter (contains some saturated fatty acid)	
"Roasted" peanuts		
Cake, pie, doughnuts, and cookies containing shortening		
All fried foods		
Animal-derived oils		

* The distinctions in this table are not absolute, but are subject to the modifications contained in the text.

What kind of oils are unsaturated? Cod-liver oil is the best. Then there are some of the vegetable oils like corn, soybean, sunflower and safflower seed oils. If vegetable oils, or any unsaturated oils, do not contain the element iodine, being unsaturated, they have the power to borrow some iodine from your system to help "activate" the saturated oils.

Then there are the oils that contain both saturated and unsaturated oils, like butter. Butter is a wonderful food, but since it contains some saturated oils, use it in small quantities. Do not use whipped butter. This makes it more saturated and less helpful to the body.

Food manufacturers add hydrogen gas to a good oil to give it a smoother texture. This further lessens its value. They do this to peanut butter, cream cheese, ice cream, vegetable and cooking oils. Oleomargarine is hydrogenated. Keep away from all hydrogenated oils. They will hurt your metabolism.

In general, vegetable and fish fats are good, animal fats not good. But we cannot say, "Keep away from all animal fats," primarily because butter is in part, good. Leaving out butter, we can say, "Keep away from animal fats such as steak fat, hamburger fat, bacon fat, sausages, corned-beef fat, salami and cold cuts, with their hidden fats ground into the meat and then colored red.

We cannot say, "Keep away from animal oils." Eggs and milk are priceless sources for animal oils. We do say, "Keep away from all oils (except butter) which are solid at room temperature. (Note that some oils, such as gravies made with meat drippings, which are liquid when served, become solid when they cool down to room temperature and therefore are to be avoided.) Keep away from chocolate candy. Keep away from cake, with its hydrogenated shortening. And keep away from all oils marked 'hydrogenated.' "

Unsaturated fish oils are needed because of their ability to pick up organic iodine. It is this ability to pick up the element iodine in the fish oils that accounts for their superior ability to repair the damage of saturated fats that keep appearing in your diet, regardless of how hard you try to keep them out. In addition, organic iodine has the power to reduce excessive amounts of cholesterol in the system. Iodine is a priceless food element.

As you can see, there is no hard and fast rule. Use your common sense. For safety's sake, start by keeping away from all solid fats.

Your body receives its supply of cholesterol from two sources: (1) from outside, via the foods you eat; (2) from inside, when it is "manufactured" by your bodily organs, mainly in your liver.

Since you can obtain cholesterol in these two ways, your only problem is to maintain the proper balance— the proper amount of cholesterol in your blood stream.

Dr. Theodore Van Italie, in the *American Journal of Public Health* (Vol. 47, December, 1957), gives three reasons why people may find themselves with an excess of cholesterol. The symptom can occur when they are gaining weight, when they are consuming relatively high quantities of fat during their meals, or when there is a disorder of the fat metabolism.

I agree. . . . That's why I have spent several years developing a dietary program and a list of menus which places particular emphasis on the correct <u>oils</u> in each meal.

Originally, my plan of diet was designed specifically for arthritics. Victims of arthritis (as well as those in danger of heart disease) must watch their consumption of oils. When the results of my dietary regimen were being clinically tested, the doctors in charge found some highly interesting facts regarding cholesterol.

Among their findings was this: patients who followed my recommended diet had <u>steadily decreasing levels of cholesterol</u>. Blood cholesterol was reduced as much as 30 per cent!

Here are some actual results, case histories:

CASE 37: Male. Degenerative arthritis and known cardiovascular complication of five years' duration.

DATE	BLOOD CHOLESTEROL
July 23, 1957	320 mg.%
October 8, 1957	270 mg.%
November 23, 1957	235 mg.%

CASE 56: Female. Mixed arthritis; glaucoma history.

DATE	BLOOD CHOLESTEROL
July 26, 1957	310 mg.%
October 10, 1957	286 mg.%
November 21, 1957	215 mg.%

CASE 66: Female. Degenerative arthritis.

DATE	BLOOD CHOLESTEROL
July 27, 1957	368 mg.%
October 1, 1957	310 mg.%
October 25, 1957	286 mg.%

CASE 72: Male. Osteoarthritis and arteriosclerotic heart disease.

DATE	BLOOD CHOLESTEROL
July 29, 1957	330 mg.%
October 4, 1957	214 mg.%
November 22, 1957	210 mg.%

CASE 108: Male. Osteoarthritis and arteriosclerotic heart disease.

DATE	BLOOD CHOLESTEROL
August 13, 1957	302 mg.%
November 19, 1957	260 mg.%
December 2, 1957	214 mg.%

The dramatic drop in the level of blood cholesterol in these typical patients was accomplished by their eating the proper foods—and by their use of cod-liver oil, a "good" oil to satisfy the body's needs, rather than a "bad" oil.

Experiments in Europe and New Proof

The value of cod-liver oil is also being tested in England and in Europe. An article in the *Manchester Guardian* (April 27, 1959) reported as follows:

Two investigators, a Dutchman and a Briton, have found that feeding experimental animals on cod-liver oil substantially reduced the amount of the oil substance, cholesterol, in the animals' blood.

Dr. A. P. de Groot of Utrecht, and Dr. S. A. Reed of Hull, put groups of rats on a diet known to stimulate the production of cholesterol, and to it were added in turn various agents which lower the cholesterol level. These included coconut oil, corn oil, cod-liver oil and various of its component fractions. Ordinary cod-liver oil proved the most effective of all the substances tested, while its "fatty acid" fraction yielded almost identical results.

Drs. de Groot and Reed were accomplishing with animals the same results which my clinical evaluation proved among human beings!

A full report was published in *Nature* magazine (April 25, 1959) by Drs. de Groot and Reed. They stated:

From numerous experiments with humans and experimental animals it is known that the cholesterol content of the blood is greatly influenced by the amount and kind of dietary fat.

In general, the relatively unsaturated vegetable fats decrease the serum cholesterol-level, while an increasing influence is observed with the relatively saturated animal fats.

The highly unsaturated oils from marine animals, however, exert a potent cholesterol-lowering activity.

A Discovery by the U.S. Department of the Interior

In October, 1959, the United States Department of the Interior released a news story to the nation's press. The headline read: RESEARCH PROVES VALUE OF FISH BODY OIL IN REDUCING CHOLESTEROL LEVELS.

To understand the importance of this subject, just read this official announcement:

> Relief for persons with high cholesterol levels in blood serum is indicated by research programs reported today by the Department of the Interior.
>
> The findings are the result of a series of research projects on fish body oil conducted by the Bureau of Commercial Fisheries, Fish and Wildlife Service, and by the Hormel Institute of the University of Minnesota operating under a Bureau contract.
>
> Bureau officials hope that their efforts will encourage clinical testing by responsible medical research staffs to evaluate the results obtained to date and to further explore the <u>application of these results on conditions which may cause or aggravate atherosclerosis and kindred diseases.</u>

(Remember, we are quoting the actual announcement by the U.S. Department of the Interior. The underscoring is mine, but the main point is the fact that a government agency is definitely aware of dietary oils. <u>They recognize that a relationship may exist between diet and heart disease, and they are urging further research in this direction.</u>

The news bulletin continued, with these vital statements:

> These discoveries were incidental to a Bureau basic research program to "take fish oil apart, molecule by molecule, and see just what it contains." Once the unique

blood cholesterol depressant effects of fish oils were noted, research programs were inaugurated to explore them. Technicians state that there is still considerable basic research needed to fully explore the properties of fish oils.

The key findings of the research are (1) the abundance of what is known as "unsaturated" fatty acids in the body oils of many species of fish, and (2) proof that the feeding of these "unsaturated" fatty acids to test animals reduced the cholesterol levels in direct proportion to the degree of unsaturation.

The term "unsaturated" in this instance applies to those fats in which there are carbon atoms which have not combined to the fullest possible extent and which are capable of uniting with certain elements or compounds to change the character of the fat.

A "saturated" fat, such as lard, congeals at low temperatures. An "unsaturated" fat does not congeal readily. This is the property which permits oil-laden fish to move freely in waters of low temperature.

Bureau research has shown that about half of the body oil of most species of fish is unsaturated and about 10 per cent of it is highly unsaturated. This latter portion of the fish oil contains five or six unsaturated carbon atoms per "chain," compared with only two such atoms in vegetable oil. In other words the potential of fish oil in reducing the cholesterol level is approximately three times that of vegetable oils.

Second only to the Bureau findings that unsaturated fish oils readily reduce the blood cholesterol levels is the development of a method to separate the highly unsaturated 10 per cent from the rest of the oil. It is this method which makes it possible to utilize only the essential part of the fish oil in reducing cholesterol levels. Thus the

patient would take only one-tenth of the calories contained in the whole oil.

The paragraphs quoted above indicate the progress
that medical science has made in controlling cholesterol,
and thereby reducing the number of heart disease
victims.

How Sugars and Starch Affect Your Heart

In addition to "oils," your daily diet must also
provide the right type of sugar and starch. If you hope
to avoid heart ailments, then pay close attention to the
carbohydrates in the food you eat.

Different forms of a food cause different reactions
on the sugar in your blood stream. The sugar arising in
the blood from eating fresh fruits and vegetables is chemically different from that obtained by eating candy.
The latter sweet becomes glucose in the same way as any
other sweet, but it is an inferior glucose which acts
differently from fruit-derived glucose, oxidizes differently, and is not valuable to the body. (It lacks critically
needed complementary factors found in whole foods that
are necessary to the full-time functioning of the body.)

This theory is in line with the findings of Dr. B. P.
Sandler. After twenty years of clinical study, Dr. Sandler
believes that the cells of the human body receive the
correct type of energy from natural sugars. He reports
that refined sugars are unnatural and even harmful.

Quick bursts of unnatural energy (derived from

devitalized foods) cause your blood sugar to rise too rapidly. This reaction is then followed by an even more drastic drop of blood sugar to levels below normal. Dr. Sandler maintains that "heart pain" and other symptoms are brought on by this phenomenon of abnormal sugar fluctuations.

For all these reasons, I believe we should avoid highly processed food and refined sugars! Many of us think of heart trouble only in terms of too much fat. Our thinking is too limited.

We should cut down on refined starches (like devitalized white bread). Instead, I recommend whole-grain breads, whole-grain cereals and baked potatoes.

To help your heart, steer clear of pastries, soft drinks, ice cream and candy. Replace these items with wholesome foods—like apples, peaches, celery and lettuce.

Even after selecting the correct foods, a person with heart disease must also be careful about drinking liquids. Again, the cardinal rule is to avoid drinking water with your meals; do not "congeal" the helpful "oils" which have to be circulated through your system. To alleviate or prevent heart ailments, you must constantly maintain the best possible circulation and combat the condition known as "blood sludge."

How To Fight the Problem of "Blood-Sludging"

All of us must one day face the problems of old age, and a common source of trouble is blood circulation.

Younger people too, become victims of "blood-sludging," so let's study this topic now, before it's too late.

To understand the dangers of "blood sludge," consider this simple definition from *Dorland's Medical Dictionary*: ". . . the clumping of red blood cells in the blood vessel system which can occur in response to disease and which interferes with adequate blood flow."

Your very life depends on an adequate flow of blood throughout your system . . . blood which will carry food values to every tissue and organ in your body.

"Blood-sludging" will prevent:

1. A normal supply of oxygen and glucose to the tissues.
2. A normal flow of waste materials and heat from the tissues.
3. Normal rates of delivery of blood to some organ (kidney, spleen, liver, etc.)

When it causes all these complications, no wonder "blood-sludging" is considered a major menace. No wonder medical scientists and nutrition experts have been working especially hard to discover an answer to "blood sludge."

Outstanding work in this field has been directed by Dr. Melvin H. Knisely at the Medical College of the State of South Carolina. He is in charge of the Department of Anatomy at the college. His years of scientific research on "blood sludge" were recognized in May of 1948, when *Life* magazine published a detailed article on his findings.

I traveled to Charleston, South Carolina, and met personally with Dr. Knisely, so that we could discuss "blood-sludging" and blood sedimentation rates. The two subjects are related, and I base this statement on the results observed when my dietary plan was tested at the medical center in Massachusetts.

The phenomena which cause "blood-sludging" also cause abnormal sedimentation rates.

Perhaps it would be helpful here if I described an actual test—how your doctor determines your "sedimentation rate." First, he takes a sample of your blood and places it in a long, narrow glass cylinder. A laboratory technician then "times" it to see how long it takes for the red blood cells to separate from the blood serum. (The red cells settle lower in the glass tube, leaving serum on top.)

Where "blood-sludging" is present in the human body, there is often abnormally fast change in the sedimentation rate. The red blood cells fall in the glass tube more rapidly; they are separating from the blood serum too quickly. This means that the red blood cells are "clumping" together, they are blocking proper circulation in your arteries.

For good health, you want the proper separation of red blood cells. You want a sedimentation rate which shows a slow settling of red cells in the glass tube.

It is definitely possible to combat "blood-sludging" by means of nutrition and your daily diet. You can lower your sedimentation rate—slow down the "clumping" of red cells—by eating the correct foods.

When my dietary plan (my list of meals and eating habits) was followed by actual patients, there was a dramatic drop in sedimentation rates. <u>Separation of red blood cells from blood serum was slower by as much as 50 to 75 per cent.</u>

This improvement in sedimentation rates—this added insurance against blood "clumping"—continued as long as the patients followed my recommended diet. The medical center reported an average improvement of 10 to 25 per cent . . . and some case histories proved three times as successful.

I have reported these findings to Dr. Knisely, with the hope that he and his associates will do further research in this direction. Proper diet can defeat the problem of "blood sludge" and can become the key weapon against heart disease.

Facts About Food To Help Protect Your Heart

We have now covered, in this chapter, the main areas of knowledge which can help prevent heart ailments. Together we have explored the value of "oils" in your diet. We have learned about cholesterol, sugars, sedimentation tests and "blood sludge."

To summarize all this information we should have a simple guide—a list of rules and suggestions—which are easy to follow:

1. Never drink water during your meals!

2. Drink room-temperature whole milk with your meals. The milk can be homogenized, raw or pasteurized, and you can drink up to one quart a day. If skimmed, powdered, nonfat milk or buttermilk are musts for you, drink them but not with the meal. Drink them about one hour before the meal, or at least four hours after eating.

3. Warm soup is certainly approved during a meal; just avoid fatty, processed, creamed soups.

4. The taking of pills (either medical or food supplements) with water can do as much harm as good if this water is taken while there is food in the stomach. Take your pills or supplements half an hour before a meal, and at least four hours after a meal. For those who must take their pills with liquid, use whole milk or soup. If skimmed milk must be used, treat it as water.

5. Refrain from drinking any iced liquids at any time. Refrain from ice cream, sherbets and any drinks containing ice cream.

6. Beer is admissible in moderation—one half hour before the evening meal or at least four hours after eating. The same schedule applies to alcohol. Never use carbonated beverages as a "mixer." It is better, in my opinion, to abstain. If taken, the drink should be mixed with water, never with ice. A better choice would be a small amount of wine, unchilled, taken one half hour before the evening meal.

7. Avoid candy, pie, cake, doughnuts, ice cream,

soft drinks and the like. Stay away from foods that provide inferior refined sugars, white flour and white rice.

8. No oleomargarine, chicken fat or roasted oils (nuts roasted in oil).

9. Avoid fried foods, potato chips and the like.

10. Vegetable cooking oils (liquid types) may be used with moderation.

11. Salad dressings should be judged on the basis of their ingredients. Olive oils, soybean oil and other vegetable oils, for example, are certainly satisfactory in moderate amounts. French dressing, with little or no sugar, and preferably wine vinegar, is permissible.

12. Meats, especially beef, are recommended, providing all visible fats are removed before cooking. (Meats should be broiled, resting on a wire mesh of some type. Never allow meat to broil in its own fat drippings. Hamburger should be lean, ground chuck or steak. Go easy on bacon and eliminate sausages and cold cuts.

13. You can enjoy an unlimited choice of fish, preferably broiled.

14. Dairy products, except highly processed foods like whipped butter, are fine, if eaten in moderation.

15. Eggs are approved, preferably soft-boiled, in moderation and if other "animal-fat" foods are kept to a minimum.

16. Use unsalted creamery butter in moderation.

17. Include in your diet soya-lecithin granules

brewers' yeast and raw wheat germ two or three times a week.

18. Use cod-liver oil mixture once a week.

19. You can enjoy an unlimited choice of foods containing high-quality carbohydrates. (Recommended are whole-grain breads, whole-grain cereals, fresh fruits and vegetables. If canned fruits are used, then drain away the syrup.)

20. There is an alarming increase in the consumption, in the United States, of Italian pizzas and Chinese foods, both of which are highly seasoned and oily in character. The seasoning produces an abnormal thirst. Americans, traditionally unaccustomed to these highly-seasoned foods, are drinking huge quantities of water, usually iced. This is one of the more recently added mistakes in our diet.

Warnings

The following seem to me to be warnings of heart trouble. Of course, no one of these alone should be considered an indication, but a number of them occurring together should be taken as a genuine indication of trouble to come.

1. Pouches beneath the eyes.

2. Yellowish lumps in the eyelids, around the eyes or in the skin surface of the body.

3. Painful sensitivity to cold air in the chest area.

4. Constipation, due to excessive intake of sweet, iced foods and the lack of foods rich in vitamin B.

5. Dandruff—too many sweets in the diet.

6. Dry or scaly skin.

7. Large pores on skin of face and ears—again a sweets problem.

8. High blood pressure.

9. Gastric distress due to overeating (belching, chronic stomach rumblings).

10. Obesity.

11. Shortening of breath, chest pain, palpitation and nervous tension.

12. Ankle or finger swelling, or both.

A CHART OF RECOMMENDED FOODS

Do your heart a favor . . . with the following foods:

BREAD
Rye, whole wheat or pumpernickel — all whole-grain breads.

VEGETABLES
All types of fresh and frozen vegetables are permitted. Pressure-cook or steam them briefly.

DAIRY PRODUCTS
Cottage cheese and all cheeses that are not highly processed — in moderation. Whole milk and small amounts of butter. Yoghurt.

CEREALS
Whole-grain cereals — whole-wheat flake cereal, brown-rice flake cereal, oatmeal and wheatmeal.

(Sprinkle on some raw wheat germ, flake-form brewers' yeast or soya lecithin granules as good dietary supplements.)

SAUCES
Only natural sauces — use no flour. Skim the fat away in meat gravies.

SOUPS
Barley soup is best. Other hot soups may be fine, as long as they are not fatty or processed creamed soups.

FISH AND POULTRY
All types of fish, including shellfish, are highly recommended. Broil when possible. All poultry allowed. Broil or roast.

NOTE: "Health foods," such as lecithin, brewers' yeast, etc., are easily obtained in health-food stores and some drug stores.

Only by an intelligent program of food nutrition can we hope to prevent the staggering loss of life due to heart disease. The total number of heart attacks is growing every year. Nearly 1,000,000 Americans died from heart ailments last year!

Even worse, today there are more than 14,000,000 people in the United States who already have some form of heart or circulatory disease.

To keep yourself from becoming a grim statistic, why not correct your eating habits? Follow a carefully planned diet; combine nutrition and common sense.

For those who are ready to try, here are a number of helpful menus.

RECOMMENDED MENUS

HELPFUL TO YOUR HEART

MONDAY

BREAKFAST

Prunes 4
Egg (soft-boiled). 1
Rye toast .... 1 slice
Butter .... ½ pat
Milk (whole milk) 8 oz. glass
Vitamin-mineral tablet
  (take with milk)

LUNCH

Tossed green salad (dressing of sunflower oil, safflower oil, soybean oil
  ... or your choice of salad dressing,
  small amount)
Cottage cheese and yoghurt
Fresh fruit
Milk (whole milk) 8 oz. glass

DINNER

Barley bean soup. 1 cup
Lettuce and tomato salad (salad dress-
  ing, small amount, of your choice)
Salmon steak
  (broiled) ...... 1 slice
Baked potato .... medium-size
Butter .... 1 pat
Milk (whole milk) 8 oz. glass

9 P.M.—11 P.M.

Fresh fruit of your choice
  (optional)

TUESDAY

BREAKFAST

Sliced orange 1
Bran and fig flake cereal
Brewers' yeast
  (flake-form) ... 2 tbsp.
Kelp granules .... ½ tsp.
Soya-lecithin
  granules .... 1 tbsp.
Rose-hips powder . ½ tsp.
  (mix four ingredients above into
  last half-portion of cereal)
Milk (whole milk) 8 oz. glass

LUNCH

Broth .... 1 cup
Sliced chicken sandwich
Milk (whole milk) 8 oz. glass

DINNER

Shrimp cocktail .. 4-5
Cucumber chunks. few
Green celery sticks several
Liver (broiled) .. 8 oz.
Melon (in season)
Milk (whole milk) 8 oz. glass

10 P.M.—11 P.M.

COD-LIVER OIL MIXTURE
  (Taken and mixed as described in
  Chapter XIII)

WEDNESDAY

BREAKFAST

Fruit or melon (in season)
Eggs (poached)... 1-2
Rye toast .... 1 slice
Butter .... ½ pat
Milk (whole milk) 8 oz. glass
Vitamin-mineral tablet
    (take with milk)

LUNCH

Consommé .... 1 cup
Fresh fruit salad
Pumpernickel
    bread .... 1 slice
Butter .... ½ pat
Milk (whole milk) 8 oz. glass

DINNER

Date and raisin salad
    (on green lettuce)
Halibut steak
    (broiled) ...... 8 oz.
Baked potato .... medium-size
Butter .... 1 pat
Banana 1
Milk (whole milk) 8 oz. glass

9 P.M.—11 P.M.

Choice of fresh fruit
    (optional)

The menus in this section will give you approximately 2,200 calories daily. About 15 per cent to 25 per cent of these calories are furnished by acceptable dietary oils.

THURSDAY

BREAKFAST

Wheat and soya cereal
Brewers' yeast
    (flake-form) ... 2 tbsp.
Raw wheat germ.. 1 tbsp.
Soya-lecithin
    granules ...... 1 tbsp.
Rose-hips powder.. ½ tsp.
    (Mix four ingredients above into
    last half-portion of cereal)
Milk (whole milk)

LUNCH

Egg (poached) .. 1
Whole wheat toast 1 slice
Butter .... ½ pat
Green salad (salad dressing, small
    amount)
Milk (whole milk) 8 oz. glass

DINNER

Onion soup ...... 1 cup
Roast beef .... 8 oz.
Beets .... ½ cup
Okra .... ½ cup
Choice of fruit
Milk (whole milk) 8 oz. glass

10 P.M.—11 P.M.

COD-LIVER OIL MIXTURE
    (Taken and mixed as described in
    Chapter XIII)

FRIDAY

BREAKFAST

Figs (black) 4
Wheat-germ flake cereal
Soya-lecithin
  granules ...... 1 tbsp.
Kelp granules .... ½ tsp.
Rose-hips powder. ½ tsp.
  (Mix three ingredients above into
  last portion of cereal)
Milk (whole milk) 8 oz. glass

LUNCH

Vegetable salad (choice of salad dress-
  ing)
Corn or rye bread. 1 slice
Butter .... ½ pat
Milk (whole milk) 8 oz. glass

DINNER

Swordfish (broiled) 8 oz.
Baked potato .... medium-size
Butter .... 1 pat
Lettuce and tomato salad (dressing of
  your choice, small amount)
Milk (whole milk) 8 oz. glass

9 P.M.—11 P.M.

Glass of milk
  (optional)

The cereals listed in the menus can be either dry or cooked
cereals, with the emphasis on whole-grain varieties.

SATURDAY

BREAKFAST

Brown rice flake cereal
Brewers' yeast
  (flake-form) ... 2 tbsp.
Raw wheat germ.. 1 tbsp.
Soya-lecithin
  granules .... 1 tbsp.
  (Mix three ingredients above into
  last portion of cereal)
Milk (whole milk) 8 oz. glass

LUNCH

Cottage cheese and yoghurt
Sliced peaches
Rye bread (toast
  optional) ...... 1 slice
Butter .... ½ pat
Milk (whole milk) 8 oz. glass

DINNER

Raisin, apple, kidney bean and celery
  salad with yoghurt dressing
Codfish or haddock
  (baked) or choice
  of lean meat.... 8 oz.
Carrots (pressure-
  cooked) .... ½ cup
Green peas ...... ½ cup
Pear 1
Milk (whole milk) 8 oz. glass

9 P.M.—11 P.M.

Green celery sticks
  (optional)

SUNDAY

BREAKFAST
Egg (soft-boiled). 1
Cottage cheese, yoghurt and raisins
Ry-krisp 2-3
Choice of berries or fruit
Milk (whole milk) 8 oz. glass
Vitamin-mineral tablet
    (take with milk)

SUPPER
Turkey salad sandwich
Carrot and celery salad plate
Dates (unsul-
    phured) 2-3
Milk (whole milk) 8 oz. glass

DINNER
Vegetable soup ... 1 cup
Mixed greens (dressing of sunflower
    oil, safflower oil, soybean oil—or
    your choice of salad dressing, small
    amount)
Steak (broiled) .. 8 oz.
Stewed fruit, small serving
Milk (whole milk) 8 oz. glass

9 P.M.—11 P.M.
2 or 3 black figs, unsulphured
    (optional)

The vitamin-mineral supplements suggested are to be those obtained from natural, organic sources—not the synthetically manufactured supplements. Often these natural vitamins have quick-dissolving substances added which make these products even easier to assimilate.

IMPORTANT NOTE: THE VALUE OF ANY SET OF MENUS CAN BE LARGELY NULLIFIED IF YOU DRINK WATER WITH YOUR MEALS. CONFINE YOUR DRINKING OF WATER TO SPECIAL HOURS. TAKE ONE TO THREE GLASSES, IF YOU WISH, ONE HOUR BEFORE BREAKFAST. OR DRINK ANY AMOUNT OF WATER YOU DESIRE AT LEAST ONE HALF HOUR BEFORE YOUR EVENING MEAL.

Chapter VII

Nutrition as a Defense Against Cancer

Fear of cancer—the fear itself, not necessarily the actual disease—is striking millions of Americans. It is a good sign when people begin to think about their health and worry about symptoms. But let's not carry it too far.

Dr. George T. Pack, associate professor of clinical surgery at Cornell University Medical School, believes that "almost everyone" has had cancer during his lifetime. "Many people live and die with cancer without even knowing they've had it," Dr. Pack said. "I would bet almost everyone has had it. I can't prove it, but I believe it's true. Man," he said, "has a tremendous immunity to cancer in his system. Somewhere in the blood stream there are immunity factors, whatever they may be, that curb cancers in somewhat the same way antibodies fight the entry of other diseases." This statement appeared in the New York *Herald Tribune,* October 9, 1959.

There have been proven cases of spontaneous regression in cancer. The course of the illness has been reversed. It has not always required surgery to stop the growth of cancer. There is hope that diet and nutrition may be able to help cause a natural regression of this dread disease.

Equally important, I definitely maintain that proper diet is a real force in <u>preventing</u> cancer. Your best insurance is to practice correct eating habits and select beneficial foods.

The very definition of "cancer" points to nutrition as the answer. *Webster's Dictionary* says cancer is "a malignant growth of tissue, usually ulcerating, tending to spread, and associated with general ill-health and progressive emaciation." Cancer is almost always accompanied by anemia and loss of strength. Food can combat this anemia to some extent, even though food alone can't cure the disease. It can strengthen the resistance, can retard the inroads. The right diet can give the cancer victim a chance. Surgery, radiation, chemo-therapy are the best presently recognized forms of cancer treatment. Check-ups with your doctor should be on a regular basis, since treatments are most effective with early stages of the disease. But I firmly believe that these kinds of intervention also need the supporting help of a proper diet, employed on a full-time year-in and year-out basis.

The most encouraging fact is, of course, that cancer has been known to <u>recede by natural means.</u> Back in 1958, a report was published in *Time* magazine concerning 120 proven cases of spontaneous regression.

I am sure that there are untold thousands of people who have had cancer without realizing it. Their bodies have automatically repaired the damage, and they have returned to good health before they were even aware of the cancerous condition. Their bodies must have been in fine shape, and they could not have been in fine shape without the right nutrition.

Radiologists sometimes take for granted their success with patients. They may fail to realize that radiation treatments also depend on the dietary background of the victim. There are certain elements within the tumor itself which decide the effectiveness of radiotherapy. For instance, the outcome may depend on the amount of organic iodine and essential fatty acids which are present in early tumor growths. This is my theory . . . and I emphasize that these elements must come through proper nutrition.

To help you combat cancer, this chapter will discuss how to assimilate "vital" foods. I will not advocate any special kind of diet. Instead, I hope to show you how to gain maximum benefit from normal meals. I will also issue fair warning against certain processed foods.

In today's food stores, we run the danger of buying too many foods which have been overrefined, overprocessed and otherwise "treated" when they were packaged. Some manufacturers add special chemicals to food—to keep it "fresh" for longer periods of time. This is known as increasing the "shelf-life" of a product. Better that the food stay on the shelf forever, than to eat some of these items!

Certain chemicals added by food-packaging companies are known to encourage cancer. I'll have more to say on this subject later. But, in direct contrast, let me cite the example of some nearly primitive people who live in Asia.

If we were to visit the Hunzas, who live today in the Karakoram region of Asia, we could learn a valuable lesson. The Hunzas are a cancer-free people. Medical researchers are discovering why. . . .

The Hunzas eat only organically grown foods. Their diet has a predominance of vegetables. They eat fresh fruits in moderate amounts. Whenever possible, their food is eaten raw. They use salt sparingly, and they have no stimulants in their diet. As a people, their weight is remarkably normal, with very few cases of obesity. They have not had a single case of cancer, and I think it is reasonable to conclude that their diet is the governing factor in this freedom from cancer.

This is another testimonial in favor of natural foods . . . and another indication that diet has a controlling effect on health. We have all heard of other instances—about Eskimos being free from one ailment, while Egyptians seem immune to a different illness. In each instance, nutrition is an important part of the answer. Diet, of course, can compensate for temperature extremes.

Cancer and Cholesterol

Now, let's become specific. Let's examine the problem of cancer, step by step. Exactly what can your diet do to protect you from this illness? The foremost advantage, once again, is related to cholesterol, in my opinion.

You will recall that cholesterol was also an enemy in the battle against heart disease. It is just as much a problem in cancer.

One of the main substances in a cancerous growth is cholesterol. *The New York Times* (January 25, 1959) reported that injections of cholesterol can produce cancer in animals. Other experiments have shown that "as cancers grow, the body produces more and more cholesterol and that the material is trapped by the tumors and probably converted to some use." Dead and decaying portions of tumors have been found to be rich in cholesterol.

These facts, stated in *The New York Times*, provide a real clue toward conquering cancer. Further evidence concerning cholesterol comes from Dr. F. E. Chidester of the Marine Biological Laboratory at Woods Hole, Massachusetts. This is presented in his book, *Nutrition and Glands in Relation to Cancer*.

Dr. Chidester maintains that dietary iodine will cause the accumulations of cholesterol in cancer to break down, thus contributing to recovery.

Too much cholesterol . . . this is the key point I am making! And how can the cholesterol levels in the human body be reduced? By proper diet!

When we found a similar situation in heart disease—too high a level of cholesterol in the blood stream —we attacked the condition by revising the patient's diet. My recommended list of foods and eating habits reduced cholesterol levels in case after case.

Therefore, it follows that if my dietary plan can lower cholesterol levels by as much as 30 per cent to protect your heart, the same meals and menus are likely to be helpful also against cancer.

Dr. Chidester emphasizes time and again that dietary oils and organic iodine are key elements in the diet for the prevention of cancer. He states that there is considerable evidence that correct diet can prevent the onset of cancer; that growth of cancer can be retarded by some diets; and that diets can help a patient to support surgery and radiation.

This expert (a Fellow of Clark University and the University of Chicago) says that "if the glands of internal secretion are functioning normally, and if the diet is adequate, there will be growth control and cancers will not normally arise." There are some important ifs there, but Dr. Chidester indicates that diet is the significant factor and I agree. (The underscoring is mine.)

Cholesterol is necessary to life. It is a carrier for oil-soluble vitamins, fatty acids and other oil-soluble factors. These latter ingredients, when available, are used for repair processes wherever needed in the body. Cholesterol is also the mother substance through which hormones are created in the endocrine glands.

It is a convenient spongelike conveyor continually in motion in the blood stream which takes into its own structure whatever oils are consumed. If the oils are good, essential ones, then cholesterol will take them where needed and they will serve their vital reparative or lubricating function. If the oil consumed is wrong and not essential, the cholesterol must still transport it and will dispose of it as energy fuel if possible, otherwise as a fat deposit. If your oil-carrier system is too busy transporting unneeded oils, it will not be able to give proper attention to the essential oils, or proper service to the needy areas. Not only will it be doing unnecessary work but it will be creating hindrances to the proper functioning of your body. This is bad enough if you are consuming enough good oil besides that troublesome bad oil. Obviously the situation is worse if you are not consuming the needed amount of good oils. Then besides overworking and clogging your system you are starving certain areas of your body.

Even a correctly balanced diet does not necessarily work smoothly with the cholesterol cycle. It is my belief that oil-free liquids taken with meals will disturb even the cholesterol transportation system of good diets. These beverages force greater quantities of the dietary oils into the liver and in turn produce a hardship on fat metabolism. Gradually, over the years, these dietary mistakes cause a rise in cholesterol. When this condition exists, the blood serum cholesterol level fluctuates. I do not think the fluctuation of even 100 milligrams in the cholesterol is crucial to the cancer problem, but it is to heart disease. When the diet is unbalanced with devitalized foods and excessive amounts of saturated or wrong fats, the process of tissue repair is seriously hampered. The process of repair depends on what substance the cholesterol is carrying in its molecular structure. If it is delivering the necessary ingredients to repair a lesion or open wound in the body, the healing or repair will proceed. If it does not deliver the necessary ingredients the lesion or wound will not heal.

Most of us visualize cholesterol disturbance playing a role limited to heart disease. Far from it; cholesterol is involved in scores of diseases. In heart disease, it is my opinion, taking oil-free liquids with fatty meals, especially iced oil-free liquids, causes the cholesterol to act in damaging fashion. Insoluble cholesterol crystals deposit themselves in the smaller coronary arteries until the passages are narrowed. The heart has to work much harder to pump the blood through these clogged arteries and is likely to become exhausted, and in the extra effort one or more of its vessels may be injured.

In cancer, the cholesterol problem is somewhat different. A diet high in devitalized foods leads to devitalized nutrition in the tissues. Poorly nourished tissues are susceptible to the formation of lesions. Persistent dieting, food additives, food colorings, chemical irritants can all do much to aggravate the lesion, once it is formed. These lesions, if not healed, can be the beginning of cancer tissue. Special reparative substances found only in the more essential foods will be needed to repair the lesion. Here is where the function of cholesterol is so important: the repair of tissue lesions before the cancer process develops.

My description of the process, simply stated, is this: Cholesterol will rush to the scene of trouble, bringing whatever ingredients it has absorbed. If it is carrying the proper wound-healing ingredients, the wound will probably heal. If the cholesterol fails to carry the needed elements, the wound will not heal, there will be an ever-increasing mass of cholesterol in the area and a tumor will probably begin to form.

World-Wide Experiments Prove Our Case

For those who still doubt whether foods are important in regard to cancer, let's travel to Japan to find added proof.

A group of Japanese investigators has studied cancer and its association with a food substance known as "butter yellow." The food industry sometimes used this substance to give fats and margarine the color of natural butter. The Japanese researchers conducted experiments with animals. They found that certain foods (rice, bran, brewers' yeast, beef liver and millet) arrested and often prevented cancer growths caused by "butter yellow."

The adding of special elements to food—to color or preserve the product—is a dangerous practice which was condemned by leading scientists at the Cancer Congress held in Rome, Italy.

Medical men from all over the world gathered in

Rome in 1956, and one topic they discussed was this threat from supposedly "innocent" chemicals. They announced that cancer may be caused by "altering" foods.

The suspected sources include the following:

Antibiotics used to fatten cattle.

Arsenic used in fruit sprays and insecticides.

Certain paraffins used for coating milk containers.

Overcooked meats: beware of charcoal-burned substances.

Certain chemicals added to chewing gum and lipsticks.

Other researchers have added more warnings to the list. They have urged us to avoid detergents that contain stilbene compounds. When dishes are washed, traces of this chemical may be left on the dishes and consumed with foods.

When you shop for groceries, read the labels and examine the package. See if you can detect the detrimental features. Learn to keep away from . . .

Meats and sausages—when treated with sodium nitrate and nitrite.

Canned foods—when treated with benzoic acid, sulphuric acid and other chemicals.

Vegetables and fruits—when sprayed with DDT and other insecticides.

Bleached flour—when treated with chemicals.

My purpose in these past few paragraphs has not been to frighten the reader. Not all processed foods are contaminated, by any means. You can still visit your neighborhood grocery store with confidence—just exercise a little more care in selecting each item.

Actually, your primary concern should be the way you design a well-balanced menu. The values you receive from good foods are what really count—the calories, the carbohydrates, the protein.

To show you how important these food values are— how they definitely affect cancer—let me tell you about a series of experiments conducted at the Michael Reese Hospital in Chicago.

Special diets were devised and fed to experimental mice, with the tests under the direction of Dr. Albert Tannenbaum. He reported these results:

1. Restriction of calories in mice on the same basic diet, considerably decreased the susceptibility to cancerous growth.
2. Further restriction of carbohydrates within the restricted diet brings about an even lower cancer incidence and at a later date.
3. Increasing the protein level of the diet from 9 to 46 per cent did not have any effect on tumor incidence. If anything, a high protein diet has a restricting effect on tumor formation.
4. Increasing the fat level of the diet caused the formation of twice as many cancerous growths

and these tumors developed earlier than those in the control group.

Throughout this book I have been naming some outstanding doctors and scientists who are actively at work seeking answers to each major illness. Here, again, in the field of cancer research, experts are studying food and eating habits.

My goal has been to write this book in simple language, to avoid complicated medical terms. I have tried to simplify the description of each experiment. For the next few pages, however, I may have to become a bit "technical." The subject of cancer is so complex that you will need to understand a few more difficult facts. So bear with me . . . and you may even find this next section more interesting.

The Role of the Pancreas in Cancer

One gland in the human body—the pancreas—has a tremendous influence in controlling cancer. According to the famous embryologist, Dr. John Beard, "When cancer cells are present in the human body, they create substances which inhibit the pancreatic enzymes which normally would be antagonistic to cancer cells."

It is my belief that iced liquids and foods cause an unnecessary strain on the pancreas, thus impeding its normal function. I further believe that laboratory tests would confirm this relationship. Avoid chilled foods and beverages and allow this very important organ to do its normal job in the war against cancer.

In view of Dr. Beard's work, it is my feeling that a person becomes susceptible to cancer when the pancreas fails to deliver certain enzymes to the body's system. Enzymes are substances which travel throughout the intestinal tract and blood stream and help "trigger" digestion, assimilation and metabolism. Without proper digestion and assimilation, the food which you eat has insufficient value.

The pancreas must deliver an adequate supply of a number of enzymes, some of which are trypsin, chymotrypsin, lipase and amylase.

Some current medical researchers now agree that cancer occurs when the pancreas is not functioning properly. This theory has been developed in detail by biochemist Ernst T. Krebs, Jr., Dr. Ernst T. Krebs, Sr., and Dr. Howard H. Beard. Their findings as stated in "The Unitarian or Trophoblastic Thesis of Cancer" appeared in the *Medical Record*, July, 1950. Much of their work was based on earlier work by Dr. John Beard.

Their findings make sense, and I'd like to add one vital fact. If your body suffers from a shortage of pancreatic enzymes, then you can do much to help your pancreas and increase the production and quality of these enzymes. First of all, stop drinking oil-free liquids with meals. Secondly, help your pancreas by adding nutritional food supplements to your diet!

It is our confirmed opinion that the best aids (in addition to a diet rich in natural foods) for nourishing your pancreas are: cod-liver oil, brewers' yeast, rose-hips powder, lecithin, kelp granules and vitamin-mineral supplements.

As you read the Recommended Menus in Chapter XX, you will note that I have included these foods as part of your dietary program for general health. However, I am convinced they are also uniquely qualified to help prevent cancer.

Eating organically grown foods [to nourish your bodily glands] is a course of action which is supported by Dr. Alexander Berglas. He is a staff member of the famous Cancer Research Foundation at the Pasteur Institute in France. (By organically grown foods, I mean foods from natural soil, fertilized only by organic or natural materials such as animal or plant fertilizer and not treated or fertilized by chemicals derived from inorganic or nonliving sources.)

Since at present it is not practical for the majority of people to insist on organically grown foods, I should like strongly to suggest that you get your foods in a state as close to natural as possible. Avoid processed, premixed and so-called "enriched" foods.

Dr. Berglas also has emphasized the role of the endocrine glands—the pancreas, the adrenals, the thyroid, etc. He, too, believes that these glands must have proper nutrition. Otherwise, they cannot function adequately and they cannot help a lesion to heal.

This noted authority describes cancer as being "a runaway healing attempt" by the body. First, according to Dr. Berglas, common lesions or wounds within the body are brought on by irritations. (The irritations may be caused by dozens of different types of chemical and food substances.) When the lesion or wound fails to heal—due to repeated irritation—then cancer cells begin to form.

Dr. Berglas has written what I consider one of the great books on cancer. It is entitled *Cancer, Its Nature, Cause and Cure.*

Nourishment for Damaged Cells

To repair damaged cells, the human body needs nourishment and all the essentials contained in correct foods. Here's my list of the food factors required:

Vitamin A: Oil-soluble vitamin A is needed for tissue growth.

Vitamin B: This complex of many vitamins is necessary to promote wound-healing and normal cellular growth.

Vitamin C: This vitamin will preserve the stability and elasticity of the connective tissue and will promote the growth of new scar tissue.

Vitamin D: Oil-soluble vitamin D will stimulate the adrenal glands. It will help localize tissue inflammation. It works best when it is accompanied by organic iodine and fatty acids (like those in cod-liver oil). It also helps

stabilize normal levels of cholesterol
within your body.

Hormones: Needed to assist in the process of
tissue repair. The hormone thyrox-
ine is particularly important. It
helps control the rate of metabolism
in the body—the conversion of food
into energy.

Protein: Indispensable for cell regeneration.

From the list shown above it is obvious that we
must include certain foods in our daily list to help
avoid cancer. By the same token, we should omit other
foods. . . . For example, stay away from white sugar!

There is growing evidence that refined starches
and sugars have a detrimental effect on health. I belong
to the group that believes that white sugar and devitalized, or "foodless" foods, are important contributing
causes to cancer. White sugar has been "stripped" of
the accessory factors which are vital to tissue nourishment. The minerals, vitamins and other key factors are
missing.

Eliminate from your diet soft drinks, all kinds of
flavored iced drinks, frozen juices, synthetic ice creams,
sherbets, refined gelatin foods and any similar food.

BY EATING WRONG FOODS, YOUR TISSUES ARE DE-
PRIVED OF NUTRIENT MATERIALS AND THEY BEGIN TO
SUFFER FROM MALNUTRITION. THIS STATE OF "MAL-
NUTRITION" LEADS TO DEGENERATION. I BELIEVE

THAT THIS KIND OF DEGENERATION CAN CAUSE A
LESION IN THE TISSUES. CANCER IS AN EXPRESSION OF
A LACK OF REGENERATION OF TISSUE!

The Value of Oxygen and "Cell Respiration"

Another area where diet affects cancer is in the
matter of "cell respiration."

The tissues of your body are composed of cells.
These cells use oxygen for respiration. If they receive
proper amount of oxygen, they will "construct" normal
tissue . . . there will be a growth of cells and healthy
tissue.

If the supply of oxygen is inadequate, the cells
become diseased and there is apt to be a growth of malignant tissue. This is not just my opinion. It is a theory
which was developed by Dr. Otto Warburg of the Planck
Institute in Germany, one of the most respected medical
scientists in the field of cancer research.

On the basis of Dr. Warburg's findings and the
opinions of other experts, I have tried to design a dietary
plan which takes into account this process of "cell
respiration." I have chosen foods and eating habits
which will help guarantee your body sufficient amounts
of oxygen.

The B-complex vitamins in brewers' yeast, and in
other foods which I recommend in my menus, help cells
to "breathe" properly. As a result, they may be crucial
factors in helping lesions to heal faster.

The action known as "cell respiration" can also be ruined by "blood sludge." This same villain we found in heart disease—"blood-sludging"—can complicate the problems of cancer. When it blocks the delivery of oxygen and nutrition carried in your blood, no wonder your cells have trouble "breathing!"

When your blood begins to sludge or slow down, a bottleneck is caused in your arterial system. Gradually, the red blood cells clump together, choking off circulation. This leads to anemia and a lack of oxygen for the tissue cells—the dangerous conditions which Dr. Warburg has listed as a prelude to cancer.

Medical examinations have shown that almost all victims of cancer also have "blood sludge." My menus and dietary plan, as you know, are designed to combat "blood-sludging." Remember too the work of Dr. Knisely (see Chapter VI). After studying 619 actual cases, he believes that increased blood sedimentation rates and "blood-sludging" have a common cause. So do I. Therefore, my recommended meals also attack this problem and help lower sedimentation rates.

Essentially, to guard against cancer, we must again follow a diet which pays special attention to "lubrication" and "oils."

We must learn to avoid all types of inferior dietary oils. Shy away from the "wrong" oils contained in bacon grease, oleomargarine, ice cream, chocolate, etc.

In addition, I suggest that everyone should take a mixture of cod-liver oil at least once or twice each month.

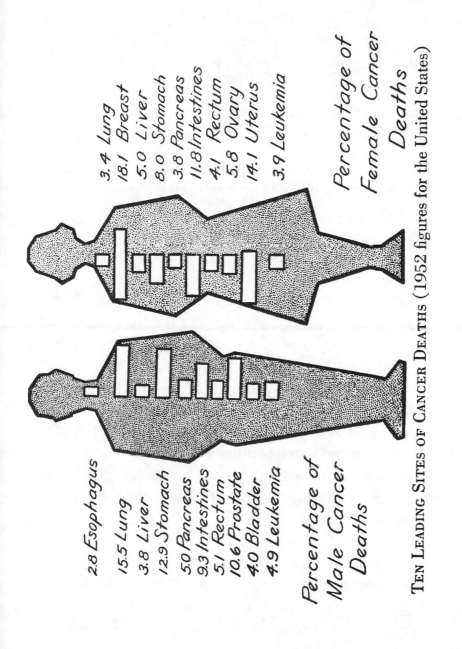

3.4 Lung
18.1 Breast
5.0 Liver
8.0 Stomach
3.8 Pancreas
11.8 Intestines
4.1 Rectum
5.8 Ovary
14.1 Uterus
3.9 Leukemia

Percentage of Female Cancer Deaths

2.8 Esophagus
15.5 Lung
3.8 Liver
12.9 Stomach
5.0 Pancreas
9.3 Intestines
5.1 Rectum
10.6 Prostate
4.0 Bladder
4.9 Leukemia

Percentage of Male Cancer Deaths

TEN LEADING SITES OF CANCER DEATHS (1952 figures for the United States)

Cod-liver oil gives you an added supply of unsaturated fatty acid. It also provides rich amounts of oil-soluble vitamin D, plus organic iodine.

Why the Same Wrong Diet Can Lay the Groundwork for Cancer Anywhere in the Body

The combination of wrong oils, overheated oils, devitalized foods, food chemicals, excessive use of salt, lack of nutritional supplements to compensate for processed foods, the lack of enzymes found in refined foods, all combine to starve or irritate the body's tissues. This will eventually produce a lesion of some kind in the body. Wherever this lesion originates, in the lung, breast, skin, bone or elsewhere, a cancer can begin.

The malnourished or chemically irritated lesion will now be at the mercy of the endocrine glands. These glands, the pancreas, adrenals, thyroid, pituitary, etc., will in turn be at the mercy of the person's diet. If the diet is poor and/or if incorrect eating habits continue, the endocrine glands cannot contribute the essential substances necessary to regulate the healing of the lesion. With healing a fiasco, the lesion area becomes a chronic, open wound.

It is at this point that the body must have nutritional supplements plus correct diet to nourish quickly the endocrines and the entire body. I believe that, lacking these essentials, the last chance for a lesion to avoid becoming a malignant tumor disappears. The cells of the lesion begin to multiply in an abnormal manner and this is cancer. The cells act as if they are rebelling against the order of nature, growing wildly.

The cells now form a tumor, or swelling. This growth gets larger and spreads through the tissues around it. It breaks them down as it continues on with its devastating invasion. Sometimes cells from the original cancer travel through the body and start a cancerous growth in an entirely different part of the body.

These cancer lesions will, I believe, more often than not, originate in organs, glands or tissues wherever there is malnourished tissue due to lack of help from the diet. Trauma—injury—could be responsible or could simply be a triggering agent when there is a background of poor nutrition.

Cancers have many properties in common. Their structures differ because they are conditioned by the strength or weakness of the host tissues.

My theory is that cancer is caused not by one single factor but a combination of many factors of which diet is of basic importance.

All of these recommendations and views are designed as protective measures against cancer.

I hope that the information in these pages may have opened your eyes to the value of proper diet, the role of nutrition as a weapon against cancer. Next, let's continue our search for better health by discussing another major ailment.

Chapter VIII

Diet Program To Defeat Diabetes

What is the fastest growing disease in America today? Not cancer, not heart disease . . . but the illness known as diabetes.

Our nation already has more than 3,500,000 diabetics. This affliction has increased by more than 160 per cent during the past twenty-five years!

How, then, can we take immediate action to reduce this terrible toll and prevent diabetes? This chapter will provide some answers, based on my personal experience with this ailment. My interest in diabetes began many years ago, when my father suffered from this condition. He had diabetes for the last fifteen years of his life. In the end, diabetic complications took his life.

One thing I remember distinctly about my father's frequent habits was his "worship" of drinking water. About five years after he came down with diabetes I asked him why he drank so much water. His answer was that he thought the more water he drank the "more dilute" his urine would be, and therefore, the less sugar he hoped to find when checking for urinary sugar.

I have never forgotten this remark of his. To me, it cost my father much unnecessary suffering. To me, his drinking water with meals was the tragic mistake of his life. I began to wonder how many other people were making similar mistakes in their eating habits. At the end, the cause of his death was cancer of the pancreas.

Later, while I was doing research on arthritis, the clinical evaluation of my diet included tests among diabetics. We had considerable success in controlling blood sugar levels and defeating other problems closely related to diabetes.

As you may know, the most important factor in diabetes is your pancreas. This body organ will determine your degree of health, and we shall discuss the pancreas in detail. You must help your body to digest carbohydrates—which supply glucose to your system. When you have diabetes, the quantity of glucose in your body increases. Carbohydrates are not being digested correctly, and the level of sugar content in your blood stream becomes too high.

To help prevent this condition, avoid drinking high-surface-tension liquids like water with your meals. In my opinion, these liquids with meals tend to "overwork" your pancreas. Refrain from drinking tea, coffee, soft drinks, flavored colored beverages, beer, alcohol and skimmed milk with meals. These are all oil-free, high-surface-tension liquids. These liquids, taken with meals, stimulate the pancreas to secrete surplus amounts of precious enzymes. This unnecessary work "weakens" the pancreas, especially if the liquids are iced.

By recognizing the symptoms of diabetes early enough, you can save yourself a great deal of grief. Why wait until you need insulin injections and other treatments? Here are "warning signs" that your pancreas is having trouble and diabetes may be developing:

Abnormal thirst
Extreme hunger
Rapid loss of weight
Easy tiring
Drowsiness
Frequent, copious urination
Itching of the skin and genitalia
Visual disturbances, blurring, etc.
Slow healing of cuts and bruises
Boils, carbuncles and other skin disorders.

Whenever a doctor suspects that his patient has diabetes, he immediately recommends that white sugar (and other sweets and devitalized foods) be eliminated from the patient's daily diet. Almost all medical men and nutritionists believe that a diabetic cannot utilize his carbohydrates adequately. Cake, candy, pie, soft drinks and all rich desserts are taboo. A person with diabetes <u>can</u> eat reasonable amounts of food containing <u>wholesome</u> carbohydrates. Among the items permitted are fruits, vegetables and the moderate consumption of properly selected breads and potatoes.

Scientific research also indicates that the pancreas of a person with diabetes contains only half as much zinc as in a healthy human being. That's why I suggest that diabetics should eat oysters, raw wheat germ, lentils and other foods which contain zinc.

Vitamins play a helpful role, too. Dr. William Brady, in his nationally syndicated newspaper column, speaks of vitamin-B complex as the "poor man's insulin." He maintains that vitamin-B complex is necessary for the metabolism of starch in the healthy body . . . to help convert starch and sugar into energy for muscular, heart and other functions.

Dr. Brady stresses that sources of vitamin-B complex are not supposed to take the place of insulin, if the patient already uses insulin. But his experience has shown that many diabetics have found that they require less insulin (to keep sugar-free or nearly so) when they supplement their diet with a daily ration of vitamin B.

I urge that a diabetic should see that his daily diet contains two or three times as much vitamin B as that of a healthy person. Of all foods, the best source of vitamin-B complex is brewers' yeast in flake form. (Brewers' yeast should not be confused with "debittered yeast"—which is a by-product of the brewing industry. Instead, make sure that you obtain primary grown food yeast. In flake form, this product has a nutty flavor.)

From brewers' yeast, your body will receive vitamin B derivatives which can help your liver carry out its functions. It will assist your liver to store starch adequately, so that the blood stream will not be flooded with sudden outbursts of sugar.

Clinical Proof of Results Due to Diet

When my dietary plan for arthritics was being tested among actual patients, the doctors in charge kept records of the sugar levels in both blood and urine. Our recommended menus and plan of eating caused marked reductions in these levels. As an indication, here are two case histories among many similar ones that could be cited.

CASE 53: A seventy-year-old male.

DATE	BLOOD SUGAR	URINE SUGAR
7/25/57	196	1 plus
9/12/57	128	trace
10/10/57	105	negative

This man was allowed moderate amounts of the proper types of carbohydrates, and a high-protein, low-fat diet. No insulin was used at any time. The only liquids permitted with meals were room-temperature milk and beneficial soups. The successful results are obvious.

CASE 1: A fifty-two-year-old female.

DATE	BLOOD SUGAR	URINE SUGAR
7/16/57	250	4 plus
8/30/57	190	negative
11/7/57	138	negative

Once this woman's eating habits had been corrected—and she stopped drinking water with her meals

—there was definite progress and an excellent recovery. She had been given Orinase simultaneously with the reglation of her diet and this undoubtedly helped, but I believe the recovery would have been achieved even without the Orinase.

Orinase, a sulfalike drug, can help against certain types of diabetes. It is effective in treating mild cases, like the type of diabetes generally found in older people.

Orinase medication (taken orally) probably stimulates the production of insulin from the pancreas or intensifies the use of whatever insulin is already in the body.

The entire subject of Orinase—and insulin—revolves around its effect on your pancreas. This vital organ, only six to eight inches long, can be your greatest asset or your worst troublemaker. Earlier researchers had learned how to isolate insulin by stimulating the pancreas with chemicals. But it was found that too much stimulation of the pancreas could cause certain parts of this organ to wear out. For this discovery millions of diabetics owe their very lives to Dr. Fred Banting and Charles Best. The research work of these two young Canadians eventually led to the synthesis of insulin, which is now used more than any other product to lower blood sugar levels.

Textbooks used in medical schools today discuss the kind of diet that should be worked out for diabetics; usually they consider how much protein, carbohydrates and fats should be in the daily diet. But they fail to specify the type of vegetables, fruits, bread, etc., which a diabetic should consume. Nor do they mention how the eggs should be cooked. (I firmly believe that a soft-boiled egg causes less strain on the pancreas than a scrambled egg.) Nor that the bread should be whole-grain. Nor do they say that the potato should be baked rather than boiled.

> **In my opinion, any diet recommended for diabetics that fails to emphasize the importance of knowing when water can be taken without taxing digestion is futile.**
>
> **It is my contention that drinking water with meals or within four hours afterward causes the pancreas to expend needless amounts of digestive juices, with ultimate breakdown of the pancreas. A diabetic pancreas at autopsy is not inflamed; it is simply worn out.**
>
> **In its own quiet way through the years, water taken at the wrong times can prove to be your worst enemy. This also pertains to any oil-free liquid.**

To help cover some of these points, let me now give you my recommended list of foods. Diabetics must keep away from the wrong kind of carbohydrates. Yet they must still maintain their weight. On page 115 are some foods which will accomplish both purposes.

Fresh fruits and vegetables should be eaten in their raw state, whenever possible. Meat, poultry and fish should be lean, and eaten in moderate portions. Breads and cereals should be of the whole-grain type only. These are the cardinal rules for diabetics. Fortunately, you can live within these restrictions and still enjoy a variety of very tasty and attractive meals. As proof, at

VEGETABLES

(any quantity allowed)

		(moderate portions)
Asparagus	Mustard greens	Beets
Beet greens	Mushrooms	Carrots
Broccoli	Okra	Onions
Cabbage	Pepper	Peas
Cauliflower	Radishes	Turnips
Celery	Spinach	
Cucumbers	String beans	
Dandelion greens	Squash	
Eggplant	Tomato	
Kale	Turnip greens	
Lettuce	Watercress	

FRUITS

(moderate portions)

Apples	Apricots	Bananas
Blueberries	Cantaloupe	Cherries
Dates	Grapes	Figs, fresh or dried
Honeydew melon	Mangoes	Muskmelon
Papaya	Pears	Pineapple
Plums	Prunes	Raisins
Watermelon	Tangerines	Spanish melon

the end of this chapter you will find a set of daily menus which will be as appealing as they are healthful.

Too many people have believed a "rumor" that diabetes is due to overeating. Nonsense! Becoming too obese does not necessarily cause a diabetic condition. In our nation, today, there are about 40 million people who are overweight. Yet our country has only 3½ million diabetics. Among the victims of this disease are 300,000 diabetic children under sixteen years of age!

Yes, people of all weight classifications are falling victim to pancreatic ailments. The problem—high levels of sugar in the blood stream—has sometimes started in childhood. But this fact should not lead us to believe that heredity is a factor. You do not inherit diabetes from your parents.

In my opinion, heredity is erroneously blamed for many diseases. What you do acquire are the habits and living ways of your parents, including their eating habits. Their favorite foods—their practice of drinking water and other oil-free beverages with their meals—become your daily routine. Too often, quite innocently, you adopt all the dietary faults that have prevailed in your family for many years.

These lifelong dietary errors are what I refer to when I list "Heredity" in Chapter I as one of the factors determining our health.

To break away from this pattern—to improve their nutritional future—diabetics can begin with the type of meals shown in the following pages.

RECOMMENDED MENUS FOR DIABETICS

MONDAY

BREAKFAST

Prunes (raw or
  stewed) 2-3
Egg (soft-boiled). 1
Oatmeal .... 4 oz.
Brewers' yeast
  (flake-form) ... 2 tbsp.
Raw wheat germ.. 2 tbsp.
  (Mix two ingredients above into
  last half-portion of cereal)
Rye bread .... 1 slice
Butter .... ½ pat
Milk (whole milk) 4-8 oz.
Vitamin-mineral tablet
  (take with milk)

LUNCH

Raw vegetable salad
Cottage cheese ... 1 cup
Milk (whole milk) 4-8 oz.

DINNER

Tomato soup ..... 1 cup
Steak (broiled) .. 4-8 oz.
Baked potato .... small
Butter .... ½ pat
Onion (raw) .... 1 slice
Milk (whole milk) 8 oz.
Vitamin-mineral tablet
  (take with milk)

9 P.M.—11 P.M.

Choice of fruit
  (optional)

TUESDAY

BREAKFAST

Sliced orange .... medium
Whole-grain cereal 4 oz.
Raw wheat germ.. 2 tbsp.
Brewers' yeast
  (flake form) ... 2 tbsp.
Soya-lecithin
  granules .... 1 tbsp.
  (Mix three ingredients above into
  last half-portion of cereal)

LUNCH

Fresh fruit salad
Melba toast ...... 2-3 slices
Cottage cheese ... ½ cup
Milk (whole milk) 4-6 oz.

DINNER

Oysters (raw) ... 4-5
Vegetable soup ... 1 cup
Broiled liver ..... 4-6 oz.
Steamed onions .. ½ cup
Tomato .... 2-3 slices
Milk (whole milk) 8 oz.
Vitamin-mineral tablet
  (take with milk)

9 P.M.—11 P.M.

Choice of celery or carrot sticks
  (optional)

WEDNESDAY

BREAKFAST

Melon in season
Egg (poached) .. 1
Rye (toast
   optional) ...... 1 slice
Butter .... ½ pat
Cottage cheese ... ¾ cup
Milk (whole milk) 4-8 oz.
Vitamin-mineral tablet
   (take with milk)

LUNCH

Choice of soup.... 1 cup
Carrots, apple and raisin salad
Banana .... medium-size
Milk (whole milk) 4 oz.

DINNER

Chicken (broiled). ¼ (small)
String beans ..... ½ cup
Brown rice ...... ½ cup
Celery sticks 2-3
Apple .... large
Milk (whole milk) 6 oz.
Vitamin-mineral tablet
   (take with milk)

10 P.M.—11 P.M.

Cod-liver oil mixture
   (Taken and mixed as described in
   Chapter XIII)

The diets recommended on these pages are designed to help your body metabolize carbohydrates correctly, and avoid wear and tear on the pancreas. However, diabetes is a disease which requires medical supervision, especially if it is beyond the early or mild stages. See your doctor regularly in regard to your insulin needs.

THURSDAY

BREAKFAST

Stewed prunes or
   black figs 3-4
Brown-rice flake cereal
Brewers' yeast
   (flake-form) ... 2 tbsp.
Kelp granules .... ½ tsp.
Soya-lecithin
   granules .... 1 tbsp.
Rose-hips powder. ½ tsp.
   (Mix four ingredients above into
   last half-portion of cereal)
Milk (whole milk) 8 oz. glass

LUNCH

Vegetable and fruit
   (combination salad)
Cottage cheese ... ½ cup
Melba toast or zweiback
Milk (whole milk) 8 oz.

DINNER

Lentil soup ...... small bowl
Roast beef (lean). 4-6 oz.
Beets .... 1 serving
Baked potato .... medium-size
Butter .... ½ pat
Milk (whole milk) 6 oz.
Vitamin-mineral tablet
   (take with milk)

9 P.M.—11 P.M.

Carrots and celery sticks
   (optional)

FRIDAY

BREAKFAST

Orange, apple, banana
(salad plate)
Egg (soft-boiled). 1
Whole-wheat bread 1 slice
Butter .... ½ pat
Milk (whole milk) 8 oz.
Vitamin-mineral tablet
(take with milk)

LUNCH

Bean and barley
soup .... 1 cup
Sandwich (salmon or tuna)
Lettuce and tomato salad
Milk (whole milk) 6 oz.

DINNER

Salmon steak
(broiled) ..... 6 oz.
Lima beans ...... ½ cup
Corn .... ½ cup
Apple .... large
Milk (whole milk) 8 oz.
Vitamin-mineral tablet
(take with milk)

9 P.M.—11 P.M.

Choice of fresh fruit
(optional)

This "Seven Day Menu Plan" lists a variety of solid foods, but only two liquids at mealtime: MILK and/or SOUP. Be sure it is WHOLE MILK and that it is served at ROOM TEMPERATURE. The soup should not be fatty or of the canned cream type. If you are seeking to gain weight, then drink more room-temperature milk at any time. Eat more sunflower and pepita seeds.

SATURDAY

BREAKFAST

Oatmeal .... 4 oz.
Brewers' yeast
(flake-form) ... 2 tbsp.
Raw wheat germ.. 2 tbsp.
Kelp granules .... ½ tsp.
Soya-lecithin
granules ...... 1 tbsp.
Rose-hips powder. ½ tsp.
(Mix five ingredients above into last half-portion of cereal)
Figs (black,
unsulphured) .. 2-3
Cottage cheese ... ½ cup
Milk (whole milk) 4-8 oz.

LUNCH

Lentil soup ...... 1 cup
Vegetable salad with parsley and watercress
Pear or apple
Milk (whole milk) 4-6 oz.

DINNER

Oysters (raw) ... 4
Lean hamburger
(broiled) ...... 6 oz.
Baked potato .... medium-size
Butter .... ¼ pat
Cole slaw
Fruit in season
Milk (whole milk) 8 oz.
Vitamin-mineral tablet
(take with milk)

10 P.M.—11 P.M.

COD-LIVER OIL MIXTURE
(Taken and mixed as described in Chapter XIII)

SUNDAY

BREAKFAST

Poached eggs on
toast 2
Smoked fish or Canadian bacon
Prunes and figs combination
Milk (whole milk) 8 oz.
Vitamin-mineral tablet
(take with milk)

DINNER

Choice of soup ... 1 cup
Broiled lean
lamb chops .... 6 oz.
Baked potato .... medium-size
Butter .... ½ pat
Tossed salad
Milk (whole milk) 8 oz.

SUPPER

Beet and egg salad
Meat or fish course
Lima beans ...... ½ cup
Choice of fruit
Milk (whole milk) 6 oz.
Vitamin-mineral tablet
(take with milk)

9 P.M.—11 P.M.

Apple
(optional)

REGARDING SNACKS: They are allowed between meals. Recommended are fresh fruit, melon in season, or any type of whole-grain food. Eat raw vegetables, with a small amount of milk. Use moderate amounts of fresh fruit, but take it easy on the dried fruits because the sugar content is too concentrated in them. No fruit juices, especially no frozen juices. Chew your fruits and vegetables well.

IMPORTANT NOTE: CONFINE YOUR DRINKING OF WATER TO SPECIAL HOURS. TAKE ONE TO THREE GLASSES, IF YOU WISH, APPROXIMATELY ONE HOUR BEFORE BREAKFAST. OR DRINK ANY AMOUNT OF WATER YOU DESIRE AT LEAST ONE HALF HOUR BEFORE YOUR EVENING MEAL. THIS PLAN WILL RESULT IN A MINIMUM STRAIN BEING PLACED ON YOUR PANCREAS. WHEN YOU DRINK WATER, THE STOMACH MUST BE EMPTY.

Chapter IX

Mental Health—The Effect of Your Diet on Your Mind

Television comedians are constantly talking about going to their "analyst" or how they live on "Miltown" to tranquilize their nerves. There's nothing funny about these "sick jokes" . . . because our nation suffers from some very real problems in the field of mental health.

To realize the seriousness of the situation, just remember these two facts:

1. Throughout the United States, half of the hospital beds are now being used by mental patients.

2. One out of every sixteen people in America is in need of some form of psychiatric treatment.

This alarming acceleration of mental illness in recent years must be halted, and I firmly believe that proper nutrition can help reverse this trend.

From time to time there are tides in the affairs of men that change our history. Almost fifty years ago there was one of those tides, and it swept one man into fame and major world importance and another one into virtual oblivion.

The almost forgotten man was Dr. Charles Mercier of London. He made careful studies of mental breakdown and came to the conclusion that mental disorders were sometimes related to mistakes in diet. He showed that diet imbalances caused mental instability and that an improvement in diet balance could bring improvement in mental health. He noted that there were excesses of sugar, starch and fat in the diets of his mental patients, and, on the other hand, deficiencies in protein, enzymes and what we now know as vitamin B.

This was in 1916, when the theories, ideas and teachings of Sigmund Freud were beginning to attract world attention. His *Psychopathology of Everyday Life* was translated into English in 1914 and the establishment, acceptance and growth of psychoanalysis stems from this time.

But at this time, in 1916, biochemistry was a young science. It had not yet been learned that sugars and starches from refined foods differ vastly from sugars and starches from natural fruits, vegetables and whole grain; that there are different kinds of dietary fats and oils, some good and some bad. Dr. Mercier was not aware of the dangers of blood-sludging or clogging, nor of the problems of blood sedimentation levels.

Dr. Mercier, because he was a little ahead of his time, failed to establish the importance of diet to mental health though he perceived this importance. His findings, incomplete and therefore unconvincing, received little attention and had no effect on medical practice or history.

The world of medicine and the world of psychology were seeking answers to the questions of mental health.

The only answers supplied were those of psychoanalysis and psychiatry. The professional world turned more and more to these for mental therapy, so that now psychiatry and psychoanalysis are fully accepted and generally regarded as the major avenues to mental health improvement.

It might have been different if Dr. Mercier could have expanded and documented his theories concerning the relation of diet to mental health. Perhaps then much more of the attention of the medical world would have been given to diet study and research, much less attention to psychoanalysis. There might have been much greater progress in the understanding of diet, perhaps much less progress in psychoanalysis.

All that is water over the dam, but it is not too late to pursue the knowledge and understanding of diet.

Dr. Louis Berman, author of the book *Food and Character*, blames mental illness on three factors: inadequate diet, unbalanced endocrine glands and poor environment.

Worry, irritability, anxiety neuroses, phobias, obsessions and compulsions . . . all these can affect the chemical reactions within your brain. These chemical reactions are, in turn, regulated by your glands. So the object is to have well-nourished endocrine glands.

How can you plan menus and meals which will be beneficial to your thyroid, adrenals and pituitary glands? Dr. Berman recommends that you should depend on a larger percentage of raw and unmanipulated foods which will provide your body with many <u>vitamins</u> and <u>minerals</u>.

My advice is stop overcooking. Stop overpreparing foods. I suggest the following foods to help <u>prevent</u> mental illness:

<u>Vitamin B</u>	Obtained from brewers' yeast, raw wheat germ, liver, egg yolk, milk, salmon, lean meat.
<u>Copper</u>	From shellfish, oatmeal, seafoods, whole grain.
<u>Manganese</u>	From beans, carrots, leafy vegetables.
<u>Zinc</u>	From oysters, lentils, liver and brewers' yeast.
<u>Iodine</u>	From seafood and cod-liver oil.
<u>Bromine</u>	From cod-liver oil.

Another expert, Dr. F. G. Hopkins, urges us to drink milk with our meals. He is the Nobel prize winner previously mentioned. Milk contains lactose—a sugar that the brain needs for its special kind of energy.

Experiments using diet to improve mental health have been under way for many years. One such test was conducted in the State Hospital at Elgin, Illinois. A group of men given yeast extracts rich in vitamin B responded favorably. When they were given a diet deficient in vitamin B, mental abnormalities increased. The successful results were reported in the *American Journal of Psychiatry* (August, 1948).

As a further example, let me cite the work of Dr. George Watson and Dr. Andrew Comrey. They published their findings in the *Journal of Psychology* (October, 1954). Here's what happened. . . .

Thirty-two patients with mental symptoms were fed a typical "American" diet. Then they were given tablets containing vitamins and minerals. The supplements used contained vitamins A, B, D, and E, plus lecithin, rutin, yeast, liver, bone marrow, alfalfa, kelp, watercress, copper, zinc and fluorine. Twenty-eight of the thirty-two patients taking the supplements showed moderate to marked clinical improvement in their mental symptoms!

Dr. Roger Williams of the University of Texas has found that individuals differ in the way they respond to food just as individuals differ in behavior. He has correlated these findings with the differences in the make-up and function of the glands in various individuals.

Some people become prone to food allergies. They do not realize that rashes, headaches, perspiration and abdominal cramps can be avoided if they know how to eat and what to eat so that full food values are gained.

Newer relationships between psychiatry and diet are being developed. Dr. Nathan Masor has written a remarkable book entitled *The New Psychiatry*. He stresses that mental illness is a problem of improper use of oxygen by the body as well as improper functioning of the endocrine glands. Here again the dangers of poor food choices and improper food assimilation can be shown.

Dr. Masor has found that the use of the vitamins B and C, thyroid extracts and nutritional supplements are of paramount importance in any mental health recovery program.

I maintain that your degree of composure can best be protected if you will learn to control your diet in regard to "blood sugar." Harmful foods (sweet drinks, rich pastries, candy) can cause drastic changes in the blood sugar level of your body. You must steer clear of any diet which will produce quick bursts of energy . . . where the blood sugar skyrockets and then quickly falls below normal blood sugar levels.

When the level drops too low, the brain reacts. You would experience weakness, tremulousness, nervous exhaustion and possibly a gnawing hunger for food. In the more advanced stages of low blood sugar, the body shows symptoms of sweating, pallor and sometimes a change in pulse rate.

If your diet is not corrected, the reactions will then be more severe. Simple nervousness may become extreme anxiety. Then you can expect to suffer from faintness, dizziness or double vision. If blood sugar levels are drastically lowered for a protracted period of time, the final result can be disorientation, confusion, and in extreme cases mania, delirium—true mental derangement.

This recital of symptoms is not listed in order to

scare any reader into believing that he is going insane. Improper food in itself will not cause a mental disease overnight. But perhaps the points made in this chapter have convinced you that your mind does need proper nutrition—just as much as the tissues and organs in the body.

Modern psychiatry is a helpful science. I have no quarrel with psychoanalysis. However, I firmly believe that recovery can be hastened—and mental damage prevented—through a sound choice of foods. Therapy should include a dietary plan.

I hope that this chapter has made one fact clear: For peace of mind, you need to understand food as well as Freud.

Chapter X

Your Eyes, Your Ears, Your Hair

From the earliest symptoms of bloodshot eyes we can fight to save our sight. Right in our own homes, we can take steps to strengthen our eyes. We can plan our meals to include foods which will safeguard our eyesight.

Yes, your eyes do depend on daily nourishment—carried by blood vessels into the retina.

I have observed the process of "eye nutrition" through a Leitz stereoscopic microscope. I have seen evidence of blood-sludging. The clumping together of red blood cells occurs in the eye, just the way it does in other organs of the body. Earlier in this book, you have learned how cholesterol deposits can clog and harden arteries in the heart. This same kind of damage can afflict the blood vessels in your eyes.

Impaired blood circulation can hasten the need for eyeglasses. The first symptom is a loss of luster in the white of the eyeball. A poor diet will also cause pouches under the eyes to grow larger and larger.

Dr. H. H. Turner, reporting in the *Pennsylvania Medical Journal* (May, 1944), maintained that carbonated soft drinks cause an abundance of carbonic acid in the system—which has a deleterious effect on the eyes. I agree. What's more, I believe that you can greatly reduce the chances of injury to eye tissues by selecting the right foods for your daily menu.

Favorable foods are readily available to help your eyes. I recommend soft-boiled eggs, milk (when you drink it at room temperature), and yellow and green leafy vegetables. Fresh fruits are suggested, if you consume them in their raw state. Rely on broiled meats, whole-grain breads and cereals. See that your body receives an adequate supply of vitamins, minerals and unrefined cod-liver oil.

We have been discussing how blood vessels nourish the retina of the eye. Now, what about the lens? The lens has neither blood vessels nor nerves. But behind the lens is a cavity containing vitreous humor, a semi-fluid, transparent substance. Many eye ailments result when this vitreous humor begins to thicken and lose its fluidity. (Cataracts occur, for example, when the lens takes on a cloudiness and becomes opaque.) These are degenerative ailments . . . and my entire dietary program is designed to combat degeneration no matter where it occurs in the human body.

An increasingly large number of individuals of all ages are wearing glasses. Thirty thousand people annually go blind. Much of this could be prevented.

Dr. Harry Eggers of New York City has found that the fat-controlling substances choline, inositol and methionine help reduce eye opacities in some of his patients. After some three years of experimenting, he published his findings in the *New York State Journal of Medicine,* October 1, 1951. He found that his patients often had increased blood sedimentation rates.

I believe that the general diets in Chapter XX can correct sedimentation rates. These better choices of foods and correct eating habits are the key.

In the case of lens-cataracts, the matter is just about decided. The cholesterol deposits are pretty well solidified. The opacities due to cholesterol deposits would be difficult to overcome. By all means, the diet should be improved immediately to accord the eyes every possible advantage in nourishing their tissues. Above all, get the diet to correct any blood-sludging and increased sedimentation rate.

Diet has to be the key. The September, 1959 issue of *Pageant* magazine carried an informative article relating diet to improved eyesight. The article points out the need for supplemental health foods like brewers' yeast, wheat germ, dessicated liver, halibut-liver oil capsules, sunflower and squash seeds, rutin, rose-hips tablets, and vitamin E.

I would prefer the use of cod-liver oil in mixture form (see Chapter XIII) in place of halibut-liver oil capsules. I also stress proper assimilation of the regular diet as well as the supplemental foodstuffs. Otherwise the eyes will not have access to the prime nourishment that the ophthalmic arteries and its branches must deliver. The eyes must be fed with proper nutrition.

Now Hear This—About Your Ears!

The threat of deafness should be enough to make us all very careful about our ears. Yet too often we ignore the early symptoms of ear trouble. For instance, have you ever bothered to check your own ears to determine whether you have a sufficient amount of earwax?

Lack of earwax is an indication that your body is "drying out," that your system needs more "oil-bearing" foods. All of the patients in our clinical study of arthritis were tested for ear maladies. They were otoscoped, and a great percentage of them had no earwax when they were first examined. After following my dietary recommendations, in case after case the patients reported that wax returned to their ears in proper supply!

Another symptom which you should heed—and act upon quickly—is "noises" in your ears. Such sounds are usually caused by inflammation, nerve degeneration or the hardening of the little bones in your ears.

The "noises" may sound like the ringing of bells, the dripping of water, hammering, or the singing of birds. Any of these can mean an inflammatory condition in your ears which will require the help of specific drugs.

If you are bothered by a "buzzing" or something that sounds like escaping steam, then I believe that your problem can be corrected through better nutrition.

Ear damage can be reversed or prevented through

special therapy which includes correct diet. This is not only my opinion . . . it has been proven by Dr. Samuel J. Kopetsky of New York City. He conducted a clinical study of 581 cases of deafness of all types. His findings are on record, published in the *Journal of the International College of Surgeons* (February, 1950).

Among the 581 patients suffering from deafness, Dr. Kopetsky consistently found that they had high levels of cholesterol. Here, again, we see that villain—cholesterol—causing real trouble in another field of health.

Dr. Kopetsky used a bland and fat-free diet—with increased protein and easily assimilated carbohydrates —to combat deafness. He also achieved results by recommending vitamin-B complex tablets combined with amino acids and trace minerals. Another of his ideas was to use fat-controlling products (lipotropic factors) containing vitamin B substances. (I believe that to gain the most benefit, you should take these supplements with milk or with soup at mealtime.)

The food factors Dr. Kopetsky recommends are available in everyday foods. Brewers' yeast contains generous amounts of choline, inositol and methionine. In addition, brewers' yeast has a large number of complementary factors. We recommend that a person who has hearing deterioration or head noises take this valuable supplement regularly.

Cod-Liver Oil Therapy Also

Dr. James A. Babbitt of Philadelphia advocates dietary treatment for hearing improvement.

In an address before the American College of Surgeons he advised dietary treatment be given only after careful study, including laboratory tests of each patient, to determine which food essentials are missing from the patient's diet.

Dr. Babbitt, quoting from another authority, said that the substitution of some foods for others—honey for white sugar, rye bread for white—improves the hearing of schoolchildren who seem to have difficulty along that line.

If this change in diet does not work efficiently within a week, cod-liver oil is added. Again, see how the need for cod-liver oil keeps coming up.

Report from the Mayo Clinic

Further evidence that one kind of deafness may be caused or complicated by cholesterol was discovered at the Mayo Clinic. At that highly respected institution, Dr. O. Erik Hallberg studied 178 cases of sudden deafness of obscure origin (i.e., not from injury or infection) over a period of five years. A report on his findings was published in the *Journal of the American Medical Association* (November 30, 1957).

Dr. Hallberg saw a pattern among the patients which indicated a connection between sudden deafness and early changes associated with hardening of the arteries.

In this kind of deafness, circulatory or sludging conditions are often present, according to Dr. Hallberg. He believes that a person afflicted with sudden deafness should be examined for symptoms of hardening of the arteries and treated accordingly. He recommends a low-fat diet. (But I believe it is more a question of "utilization" of what you eat—rather than a low-fat diet. The latter is not the full answer to the problem. And there are two kinds of utilization to contend with: initial, as you eat, and secondary, blood-sludging interferences.)

How can you tell whether your present diet is affecting your ears? Well, one danger sign is an attack of dizziness. If it occurs repeatedly, then chances are that your diet is not being properly digested and assimilated. Blood-sludge may be causing inadequate utilization of your food. When too little blood is being delivered to the cochlea and equilibratory labyrinth in your ears, then you will experience dizziness.

Ask your own doctor about the present condition of your ears. After he examines your ears with an otoscope (an ear mirror), discuss with him the subject of earwax. Is there wax present? What color is it—what consistency—what quantity? It should be yellow, of an oily consistency. (In some cases due to changes within the ear structure, even correct diet will fail to secrete normal supplies of earwax.) If none is present, are your ears itching too often? How long has the ear been dry?

These questions are your "check-list" . . . an easy way to anticipate ear ailments and prevent them!

Food for Thought Concerning Your Hair

As we seek to improve our health through better nutrition, we should regularly examine our hair. A normal scalp and a continuing growth of hair are indications of a sound body condition.

By the same token, if you are having problems with your hair, that may mean that your entire system is in danger of more serious disorders and ailments. Your scalp can show symptoms of "malnutrition" and warn you in time to prevent a major disease.

Never minimize what may seem to be only minor troubles involving your hair. Check yourself today for any of the following conditions:

1. Persistent dryness of the hair and scalp.
2. Scaling, and the presence of dandruff.
3. Itching sensations, or a particularly tender scalp.
4. Thinning, increased presence of loose falling hair in your comb or brush.
5. Recession of hair at the temple line.

6. A pattern of baldness, beginning at the top of the head.
7. Excessive oiliness of the hair and scalp.

The relief of many of the above annoyances can often be found through proper diet. The major requirements for proper hair and scalp health are vitamins (especially vitamins A and B), germinating factors, oils, minerals, pigment and protein.

Vitamins and Foods to Increase Growth

Many doctors recommend diets to stimulate the scalp and the growth of hair. Dr. Herman Goodman, a leading dermatologist in New York City, suggests foods which are rich in vitamin A. He is the author of *Your Hair,* and he favors menus that feature raw, fresh eggs and carrots.

Dr. Richard W. Muller's experience and practice in Paris, London, Vienna and Berlin have caused him to rely on foods which contain plenty of sulphur. Raw milk and oatmeal are also effective. The iron in eggs can be beneficial—iron is an important element in hair.

Dr. Muller emphasized that calcium also is an important hair component, and we should eat meaty soups and bone-meal powder for this element. I know that rye bread can also help build our supply of minerals.

For better hair health, I urge that you eat a soft-boiled egg two or three times each week. Have raw car-

rots once a week. On another day, every week, try carrots that have been pressure-cooked briefly.

A person who suffers from chronic constipation
is likely to have subnormal hair growth. This medical
opinion comes from Dr. Oscar L. Levin and Dr. Howard
T. Berman. Their book, entitled *Your Hair and Its Care,*
explains the relationship between constipation and scalp
diseases. They recommend meals which do not contain
any sweets or white sugar. (This is plain common sense.
I maintain that too much dimineralized white sugar is
one cause for the lack of needed minerals in your hair!)

Your system must produce adequate amounts of
melanin pigment or coloring matter for the cortex of
the hair. And you must prevent air bubbles from collecting in the middle layer of the hair. Both of these goals
can be accomplished through proper diet.

The question of pigments (like melanin) was explored by Dr. Franklin Bicknell of French Hospital in
London, and by Dr. Frederick Prescott, clinical research
director of the Wellcome Foundation. These doctors
agree that ascorbic acid (vitamin C) inhibits the formation of pigment.

Explained more simply, to prevent gray hair and to
improve pigmentation, you should reduce your consumption of certain fruit juices which contain too caustic
a type of ascorbic acid.

To avoid "dryness," lubricate and nourish the hair
shaft with a dietary oil which is rich in vitamin A and
iron. The best choice, again, is cod-liver oil.

Nutrition's Role Against Baldness

Digestion and eating habits are closely related to abnormal loss of hair. This fact has been proven medically, and one example is the work of Dr. Lucien Jacques, a leading dermatologist. He conducted an experiment, at the Saint Antoine Hospital in Paris, involving 71 patients who suffered from gastrointestinal disorders. All of these patients were also losing their hair too rapidly.

Dr. Jacques found that the majority of the patients ate too fast and did not chew their food well enough. Therefore, food substances were not mixing properly with saliva secretions. The patients also drank excessive amounts of tea, coffee and alcoholic beverages with their meals.

Dr. Jacques changed their diet. According to his clinical report, his changes produced remarkable changes in the health of the hair! When indigestion was overcome through better eating and drinking habits, the hair loss ceased to be abnormal, new hair grew and the general health improved.

Progress in preventing baldness has been demonstrated by many other nutritionists in recent years. My own experience—the observations made during the clinical tests on arthritis—showed that hair will respond to correct diet. Incidentally, the clinical study on arthritis (described in Chapter XXI) revealed a surprising fact about women. Thinning hair is a far greater problem among women than is publicly acknowledged. More than 80 per cent of the patients studied were women. The majority of them had either dandruff or thinning hair. Some had a considerable hair loss—until they adopted my menus and dietary program.

The oil-bearing diet plus sprouting foods and strengthening food supplements is your guide to forestall baldness, to lubricate your scalp and to encourage lustrous hair.

These diets cannot be expected to restore hair. However, in many years of observation I have noticed that where such foods as onions, scallions and garlic (sprouting food, necessary for the germinating layer of the scalp) are important items of diet, more people retain their hair. More of these foods could be used in salads in the menus. For those who find ordinary onion too strong, the red Spanish onion is milder. Raw wheat germ also has been found beneficial and is an excellent food for the germinating cells of the scalp. All these foods are useful in nourishing the scalp and hair. But don't undermine their benefits with sweets. Remember, white sugar, sweets of the refined type like ice cream, sherbet, soft drinks, pastries, candy, etc., are especially bad for the scalp and hair. If you want healthy hair, keep away from devitalized, processed foods. Increase your choice of the natural foods. It is most important that you do.

Chapter XI

Diet Versus Dental Decay

Your dentist is a guardian of your health to a far greater extent than you may realize. When he discovers cavities and other problems of the teeth, listen to his warnings and advice. Dental research has proven that often diseases of the body are related to diseases of the mouth.

So let's examine the cause of toothaches, decay, etched teeth, pyorrhea, gum erosion and gum recession. Let's discuss the value of trace minerals—like fluorine, magnesium, iodine, boron, cobalt and copper. These elements, in a balanced diet, are your best protection against the dental troubles mentioned above.

To explore this subject in more detail, I would like to report on the work of four doctors, pioneers in the field of dental research. The group includes Dr. Weston Price of Cleveland, Dr. Melvin Page of St. Petersburg, Dr. George Heard of Hereford, Texas, and Dr. Harold Hawkins, who was formerly associate professor of preventive dentistry in the College of Dentistry, University of Southern California. They all recognized the importance of correct diet in relation to teeth. Each wrote a book revealing the results of his research. Here is my summary of some of their findings. . . .

1. To have strong, healthy teeth, we should include in our meals raw vegetables, natural grains, fruits and foods grown in organically sound soil. We should also depend on wholesome dairy products (like raw milk) and the organs of animals (like liver).

2. Raw milk was recommended over pasteurized milk. "Milk drinkers live longer and stay younger for their age than non-milk drinkers. They suffer less from dental caries and arthritis . . . and as a class they are less nervous and suffer less insomnia."

3. The experts were against fruit juices, but favored raw, fresh fruits (chewed well).

4. Cod-liver oil was recognized as a good weapon to help arrest dental decay. To contribute hardness to the teeth, these dentists urged us to rely on trace minerals—including fluorine.

The four major points which I have just outlined represent my composite version of the opinions of these four doctors. And right now I would like to state my own position on the controversial issue of fluorine.

Fluoridation—adding chemicals to the water supply in your city reservoir—may have caused a great debate in your home town. Newspaper headlines have been made in many areas by dentists and other medical men who have campaigned in favor of fluoridated water.

I realize the value of fluorine, and recommend it to strengthen teeth. However, I am opposed to tampering with city water supplies. Why add fluorine by artificial means, when it is already available in several natural foods? The simplest way for your body to gain an adequate supply of organic fluorine is to take cod-liver oil. Just follow the menus—and cod-liver oil plan—described in this book (Chapters XX and XIII).

Organic (animal or plant) fluorine (as in cod-liver oil) is particularly essential to a woman during pregnancy. It has been found that the placenta of a pregnant woman can filter fluorine from the blood stream and pass it on to the unborn child. The baby will then have a better chance for fine teeth, and the mother herself will experience less dental decay.

During each pregnancy, my wife took cod-liver oil once a week. Later, our children were given vitamin and mineral concentrates. Today our son Dean is ten years old. Our daughter Joan has celebrated her sixth birthday. Neither has ever had a single cavity!

Our children continue to take a cod-liver oil and orange juice mixture about once a month. The purpose is to make organic fluorine and oil-soluble vitamins available to harden their teeth continually. This oil-soluble vitamin D also contributes calcium and phosphorus—helpful to the enamel of their teeth.

Adults, too, would do well to follow these same suggestions. With a little common sense you can greatly reduce your dental problems throughout your lifetime.

Why "Primitive" People Have Better Teeth

Perhaps the most extensive research in the history of dentistry was accomplished by Dr. Weston Price when he traveled around the world to study the living habits of primitive people. He took thousands of photographs of their teeth, jaw structures, facial contours.

Dr. Price and his wife visited and collected data among the Eskimos of Alaska, the Polynesians and Melanesians in the South Pacific, the aborigines of Australia, the Maoris of New Zealand, the natives in Africa, the jungle folk in Peru. Throughout his journey, he found entire groups of people with strong, hardy teeth. Why? What caused their dental superiority over modern Americans?

The eating habits of those "uneducated" people were basically the same—and in many ways they were far wiser in their choice of foods than we are today. Their diets included an abundance of seafoods—fish chowders, cod, lobsters, oysters and clams. When eating animal meats, they preferred liver, heart and kidney instead of the muscle meats. They consumed bone marrow. Grains were eaten whole—never milled or refined. Fruits were chewed, not liquefied into juices.

When explorers and settlers visited these native tribes, they brought with them white sugar, white flour and other processed foods. When the primitive peoples adopted such foods, within one generation their dental health began to deteriorate.

Children developed tooth decay. There were changes in the dental arch, "crowded" teeth, a narrowing and lengthening of the face structure. Dr. Price brought home photographic proof of these afflictions, and traced their cause to the advent of "modernized" foods.

CIVILIZATION HAS MANY ADVANTAGES, BUT ALSO SOME DISADVANTAGES—PARTICULARLY IN RELATION TO NUTRITION.

Watch carefully your consumption of refined foods, and remember that white sugar can disturb the balance between calcium and phosphorus within your body. Calcium and phosphorus, properly balanced, make "carbonate apatite." This is the mineral compound of which tooth enamel is composed. A deficiency in this compound will cause a deterioration or weakness in your tooth enamel.

Demineralized sugar can also cause a deficiency of vitamin B in your body. Vitamin B affects the level of ptyalin in the saliva. Without enough ptyalin in your saliva, acids will attack the structure of your teeth. To increase your ptyalin level, it's advisable to augment your diet with brewers' yeast, raw wheat germ or both.

The Dental "Miracle" in Hereford, Texas

Any chapter about our teeth—any discussion of "Look Ma, No Cavities!"—should include some facts about the sensational case of a little town in Texas. There have been too many rumors and not enough truth about what actually happened in Hereford, Texas, a few years ago.

You may remember the newspaper stories which

told how the population of Hereford was remarkably immune from cavities.

This community in Texas became the center of a nationwide controversy between the "pros" and "cons" of fluoridation, due to the work of one dentist. Dr. George W. Heard, who practiced dentistry in Hereford for some twenty years, deserves credit for awakening the entire country to this phase of dental health.

Dr. Heard was impressed by the low rate of dental decay in his area of Texas. He believed that this was true because of what people ate, the kind of milk and water they drank, and the type of soil that produced their food.

In cooperation with Dr. Edward Taylor, director of dental health for the Texas State Board of Health, Dr. Heard conducted a large-scale examination among the residents of Hereford. The results showed an almost complete lack of dental decay, and this discovery was reported to the American Dental Association.

Somehow, newspapers and national magazines jumped on the idea that the drinking water in Hereford was mainly responsible for these thousands of cases of strong, healthy teeth. Prematurely, they credited this dental success story to the amount of fluorine in the drinking water.

The fact that Hereford had 2.2 parts per million of fluorine in its water supply (compared to 1.9 and lower amounts in the surrounding towns) is how the mistaken idea grew that fluorine in the water made the difference.

Many public groups throughout America began to clamor for this same type of "protection." "Add chemical fluorine to our local water supply!" they said.

This would make sense except for one fact. There are two kinds of fluorine—inorganic (from mineral sources) and organic (from animal or plant sources). If a city adds inorganic fluorine to water, too much of this substance can be a real danger. Inorganic fluorine is a known poison. Excessive amounts can mottle the teeth, rather than improve them.

Organic fluorine is beneficial. Gain your requirement of fluorine from foods! Properly grown wheat products contain some 400 parts per million content of organic fluorine. This far surpasses the amount of fluorine in ordinary drinking water.

Soil rich in minerals, including fluorine, can impart this element into foods as they are grown. Therefore, you can receive fluorine from wheat, corn, carrots, turnips, potatoes, cabbage, green beans and lettuce.

Dr. Heard himself later wrote a book, in which he emphasized that inorganic fluorine in water is not responsible for sound teeth. Fluorine in water is not a food and, consequently, it is not utilized by the body. He feels that "the right combination of elements in the soil, when taken up by food plants and then consumed as nearly as practicable in their raw state, will prevent tooth decay."

You now have read the <u>true</u> story of Hereford, Texas. Just remember that no single mineral and no single vitamin will build perfect teeth.

Basic Dietary Needs for the Teeth

The work of the pioneer dentists mentioned before is being taken up by current dental researchers. Dr. James H. Shaw, associate professor of biological chemistry in the Harvard School of Dental Medicine, writes an interesting chapter in the book *Modern Nutrition in Health and Disease*. In the section entitled "Nutrition in Relation to Dental Medicine," he writes:

> The best advice for any age group about the dietary regimen that will provide the best opportunity for normal oral tissues is simple and straightforward. Each of the basic seven * food categories should be represented liberally in each day's diet, and as many as possible in each of the day's three meals.
>
> The best selections of food for dental health is one where as many of the foods as possible are purchased in their natural state without excessive refining and where the cooking procedures are such as to conserve the maximum of the original nutritive value. Attention should also be paid to the inclusion in the diet of a frequent and varied series of foods that require vigorous mastication as a means to stimulate and exercise the various tissues and organs involved in the comminution [grinding] of food. In addition, a liberal source of vitamin D should be provided daily throughout the entire period of

---

* Dr. Shaw's "categories" are classifications of a different order from my "categories," which are: proteins, carbohydrates, fats, vitamins, minerals (the standard five) plus water.

an individual's growth and development. A minimum
of sticky, adherent, high-carbohydrate foods with a low
rate of clearance from the oral cavity should be consumed. After eating foods with a slow oral clearance,
the teeth should be cleaned thoroughly by the procedure
of choice to be recommended by the dentist. As in-
between-meal snacks, in place of sticky high-carbohydrate foods, fresh fruits, vegetables, fruit juices, milk
and other dairy products are much to be preferred from
a dental health standpoint. In the over-all nutritional
planning for improved dental health, one of the most
important facts to be considered is the fluoridation of
public water supplies." [As noted earlier, I believe the
fluorine in cod-liver oil is far superior, and more natural
for the maintenance of teeth and bone.]

Most of this chapter has been devoted to the cause
and prevention of dental decay, but what about your
gums? They are an important reflection of your general
health. If your gums are not as they should be (solid,
and a pink color) it is safe to say your body is in need
of dietary improvement. Unhealthy gums (spongy,
bleeding, poor color), generally indicate nutritional imbalance elsewhere in the body. What do we base this
on? Dental literature and common sense. It is common
knowledge that it is perfectly possible to have sound
teeth, with or without fillings.

Vitamin C is an important factor in health of gums.
In our opinion, whole fruits, which must be chewed, are
better than any form of juice. I am opposed to the use
of fruit juices, especially frozen.

Dentists Versus a Mountain of Cavities

According to Dr. Fred Miller, a practicing dentist in Altoona, Pennsylvania, who specializes in preventive dentistry through proper nutrition, dental decay is the most prevalent disease known to civilized mankind. At least 98 per cent of the population of the United States suffers from dental decay. He reports that exhaustive surveys by the American Dental Association indicate that there is a backlog of over half a billion cavities in our country. Dr. Miller feels that dentists cannot possibly keep up with the increase of dental decay, to say nothing of the other dental diseases, which include destruction of the bony support of the teeth and diseased gum conditions. Filling the cavities is not the answer, according to Dr. Miller. Dentists and people must strike at the cause. He adds that controlling dental decay and destruction of the gums must be done through a sound nutrition program.

My answer is a complete nutritional program . . . a diet of foods grown in properly nourished soil. The addition of cod-liver oil (mixture form with either milk or a very small amount of fresh orange juice) is tremendous insurance for the prevention of teeth and gum troubles. I believe the cod-liver oil part of the program is the key.

Organically grown foods plus cod-liver oil are the only safe and sure means to check degeneration within the mouth. Having learned the right way to achieve healthy, attractive teeth . . . keep smiling!

Chapter XII

Some Advice on the Common Cold

"Feed a cold and starve a fever" is a folk saying that gives recognition to the important relationship between diet and the common cold.

Susceptibility to common colds begins through wrong nutrition. Of course, insufficient or faulty nutrition makes you vulnerable to many ailments, but in the case of colds the factor is greater simply because there are so many cold-carriers and they are almost everywhere.

Obviously, then, to protect yourself from colds it is wise to watch your diet and be sure your body is getting the right nutrition to maintain its strength. But apart from this generalization, there are certain specific dietary steps you can take to defend yourself against colds.

Dr. Alexander Fleming, who earned a Nobel prize for his research on penicillin, discovered that a substance called "lysozyme" is present in various secretions like saliva—and that it has the power to break up and disperse certain bacteria. We now know that bacteria can be rendered harmless by the presence of lysozyme in the nasal secretions. We also know that a sharp reduction of this substance in the nasal secretions is an indication that you are catching a cold. Conversely, if you have a cold there must have been insufficient lysozyme in your nasal secretions.

Tests made at Columbia University in New York proved another key fact about lysozyme. These later experiments showed that the bacteria-dissolving powers of lysozyme could be increased by as much as 250 times through the addition of minute amounts of biotin.

Your best food source of biotin is brewers' yeast. Biotin is one of the many vitamins of the B-complex. By adding brewers' yeast to your diet, you can build up a stronger resistance to temperature changes—chilling rains and snow, poor air-conditioning systems, ordinary household drafts. Naturally, I recommend brewers' yeast.

For many years, doctors believed that colds were related to bacteria. Recently, the emphasis has changed from "bacteria" to "virus." But "bacteria" or "virus," the mechanism by which we catch colds is still the same.

Yes, I recommend vitamins to help prevent colds. Vitamins A, B and C are most helpful. Vitamin C (as ascorbic acid) can unite with cholesterol in your body and will produce protective hormones. These hormones will keep your resistance to colds at a high level and will minimize any drastic circulatory changes.

In your effort to gain vitamin C, however, don't rely on juices. When you drink fruit juices, you rush massive amounts of acid into the system without sufficient neutralization by the saliva. Enjoy whole fruits . . . eat that orange or tomato . . . and chew it well. If you feel that you are highly susceptible to colds then you should consider using vitamin C in a more concentrated form. But don't make the mistake of relying too much on grapefruit or lemons. These are too caustic, therefore less desirable than oranges. Add some rose-hips powder to your menu or take acerola tablets for greater amounts of vitamin C. Take these two health food products with milk.

Oil-soluble vitamin A (as found in cod-liver oil) can make a valuable contribution toward preventing colds. Your anticold diet will also benefit from green and yellow vegetables.

Know Your Nose

Any discussion of the common cold should include the pertinent facts about your nose and your nasal passages. Too many people do not understand the vital function of this part of our anatomy.

The nose serves as a "humidifier" and "air-conditioner." It filters and regulates the temperature of the air we breathe. The mucous membrane in the nose supplies moisture to the air we inhale.

How You Trigger Your Own Cold

We are surrounded by germs. We keep breathing them in all the time. Most of the time they have no effect on us, but sometimes they catch hold, stay in our systems, and we have a cold or a disease. What are the conditions that are favorable to germs and therefore unfavorable to us? Germs need something to feed on, they need a host. If they have nothing to feed on, they will not get into your system. What do they feed on? Devitalized sweets like chocolates, syrups, white sugar are the favorite food, the natural hosts, of germs.

If you eat some chocolate during a meal and then consume other foods and liquids which carry the chocolate down so that they do not linger in the throat, the danger is much reduced. However, if the chocolate or similar sweet is consumed at the end of the meal, as is customary, it is likely to linger in the throat. In addition to thus being available to germs, these sugary particles irritate the mucous membrane of the respiratory tract and disturb for about twenty minutes the film of mucous that covers the membrane. This lowers your resistance and increases your vulnerability. And the vulnerability continues for a little while, even after the particles of food have passed along. During this period cold germs are much more likely to affect the irritated mucous membrane. If a cold-carrier is nearby, or if you are in a draft, or the weather is inclement, you are likely to catch a cold, whereas someone who has not eaten sweets is not so likely to be infected.

For this reason, if you are fighting a cold, beware of items like chocolate, cookies, all types of cakes, ice cream, sherbet, glazed doughnuts, etc.

Perhaps colds are more prevalent because it is

customary to end a meal with such sweets. The child who has a cookie or a piece of candy continually in his hand is a prime candidate for a cold. It is my theory that we induce our own colds by the frequency with which we permit ourselves to have sugar residues in our throat.

Prevention

It is common sense to attack the common cold before it gets started. Let's learn to use proper nutrition—natural foods—as a means of prevention. To help you build your resistance, here is a list of recommended rules:

1. Keep away from syrupy candies, chocolate, frostings, sweets of all descriptions when in the presence of anyone who has a cold and especially if you have a cold.
2. Through more fruits and vegetables in your diet, add to your natural supply of vitamin C. Eat salads more often.
3. Build up your supply of oil-soluble vitamin A. Good food sources are soft-boiled eggs, room-temperature milk, butter and cod-liver oil.
4. Avoid lemonade and acid fruit juices when trying to cure a cold. Instead, try soup or broth. Barley or bean soup, or vegetable stock containing plenty of greens, is excellent. Get plenty of rest, go to bed and recover.

5. If you suffer from chronic colds (or asthma or hay fever allergies) use no wheat products that are refined. Your best bet is to eat rye or dark breads, and use organic wheat products.

6. Increase your intake of the B-complex vitamin known as biotin. Add brewers' yeast to your menu. Or gain vitamin B through yeast in powdered or granulated form.

7. Keep regular. Depend on natural foods to avoid constipation. (See Chapter XVIII.)

The above list of seven suggestions is a simple summary of my entire program to prevent and relieve the common cold. You now have a dietary defense against this annoying illness.

Now, however, let's turn to a more painful ailment . . . let's discuss a crippling disease which affects more than 11,000,000 victims throughout the United States.

Chapter XIII

The Leading Question: "What About Arthritis?"

My answer to arthritis problems has led thousands of people to relief from pain . . . and has led me into the center of a stormy controversy with the medical profession.

I have been praised and thanked by victims of arthritis throughout the United States. Simultaneously, I have been attacked and condemned by certain doctors who refuse to believe that diet can help arthritics.

The details of this great debate will be discussed more completely in Chapter XIV. But right now let me state one basic fact. Despite all criticism—all the pressures brought to bear against me during the past 15 years—I have not changed my original concept. I still believe:

"You can eat your way into arthritis . . . and you can eat your way out!"

Now, in two or three paragraphs, let me summarize my theory about arthritis.

All we have to do is to look at the definition of the word arthritis. The prefix "ARTH" means joint. The suffix "ITIS" means inflammation. Compounded, ARTHRITIS means "inflammation of the joint."

What causes this inflammation?

FRICTION causes bodily joints to become inflamed. If the "oils" in your body dry out, the joints begin to "creak." The surfaces of the joints rub against each other, and a grinding action sets in. The bony structure becomes damaged . . . and the whole area becomes swollen and inflamed.

There, described in a few words, is the cause of the most prevalent kind of arthritis, osteoarthritis. Rheumatoid arthritis involves the stiffening and inflammation of other tissues also.

The best method to reduce the swelling in arthritic joints, to ease the stiffness and to lessen the pain is to "lubricate" your body internally. Dietary oils—obtained from the foods you eat—can do the job.

To increase the flow of "lubricating oils" throughout your system, I have devised a series of special menus. Some of them are listed later in this chapter. I have developed a list of recommended foods, which you will find in this chapter. And I have suggested that arthritics should augment their diet of "oil-bearing" foods by taking specified amounts of cod-liver oil. In essence, you have now read my entire plan of action against arthritis.

Sounds simple, doesn't it? In fact, you might be tempted to ask whether such an easy solution can be really effective? In reply—to prove that diet can defeat arthritis—let me tell you the inside story of a certain television show.

Perhaps you have seen the TV program about arthritis, during which Conrad Nagel interviews me and asks probing questions about my theories on diet. This particular telecast has been shown in more than 100 cities across the nation. Now, let me take you behind the scenes and show you how this TV film was made. I'm referring particularly to the "conference room" sequence which impressed millions of viewers. Sitting around a conference table were four people who had been victims of arthritis, ready to tell their experiences after they had read my book.

Some weeks earlier—before the film was to be made—I had received letters from these four arthritics. They wrote to me, like thousands of others, to report how successful my diet had been for them.

For many years I have been receiving unsolicited mail from grateful men and women everywhere, reporting that my dietary plan does work. When it came time to make a TV film about arthritis, we merely selected four typical case histories.

After reading their letters, we telephoned these four people at their homes and told them that a TV film was going to be produced on the subject of arthritis. They offered to come to New York and appear in the motion picture—without any payment whatsoever for their services or their endorsement of my book.

I repeat, these were not paid testimonials. All of these people—from various walks of life—were sincerely grateful for the help they had received from

Arthritis and Common Sense. They volunteered to tell millions of TV viewers about their successful fight against the disease.

Before the people arrived in New York, their original letters to me were read again and then written into script form. Since these people were not professionals it was felt they would need a script to follow as a guide.

Then came the day of the filming, and a surprising incident. . . .

The four guests sat down at the table with Mr. Nagel and me. To set everyone at ease, the director suggested that everyone "just talk about arthritis" while the microphones were being tested and cameras set in place. It would be an "ad-lib" rehearsal.

When these four arthritics began to talk, the camera crew was amazed. They were so enthusiastic—so sincere in their discussion of the book—that no script-writer could have matched their dialogue. So the script was thrown away! The cameras were turned on, and this is what these typical arthritics said . . . in their own words. . . .

ACTUAL QUOTES FROM THE SOUND TRACK OF THE ARTHRITIS TV PROGRAM

CONRAD NAGEL

The first of our guests has traveled from Galesburg, Illinois, and is Mrs. Russell Watson. Mrs. Watson, just when and where did arthritis first strike you?

MRS. WATSON

I have had arthritis off and on for the greater part of my life. But about three and a half years ago it settled very badly in my neck and shoulders and arms, and then went all over my body.

CONRAD NAGEL

Well, after reading the book and following the instructions, how soon did you notice an improvement?

MRS. WATSON

I noticed improvement in the first few weeks, and after about six weeks my pain was entirely gone. And after about a year I was completely well!

(*Next*, MRS. OSWALD JACOBY *of Dallas, Texas*)

CONRAD NAGEL

Mrs. Jacoby, how long have you suffered from arthritis?

MRS. JACOBY

I have suffered for eight years in the cervical and lumbar regions of my spine. Several months back it traveled to the base of my spine. At that time my husband brought home Mr. Alexander's book from Memphis. I read the book and followed his dietary regimen rigidly, and within two weeks the pain had left the base of my spine.

CONRAD NAGEL

Did an over-all improvement continue?

MRS. JACOBY

Definitely!

(*Next*, MR. ROGER VREELAND, *newspaper editor, from Paterson, New Jersey*)

MR. VREELAND

I found arthritis a very definite handicap in my work. In fact, my fingers were so bad that I could hardly pound the keys of the typewriter, and as a matter of fact, I could hardly hold a pencil. From my hands it moved to my feet. The doctor diagnosed it as rheumatoid arthritis, and for many years I had to use a cane. I started [following Alexander's dietary plan]. And within two to three weeks the pain left me, I felt very much improved, and from then on the progress was steady.

(*Next*, MRS. MARGARET MILLMAN *from Plymouth, Mass.*)

CONRAD NAGEL

Was your problem with arthritis at all similar to the others we have heard from?

MRS. MILLMAN

Yes, Mr. Nagel, somewhat similar. I had arthritis in the terminal joints of my fingers. I also experienced considerable stiffness of the hips upon arising. This condition had been developing over many months, and since it was becoming worse I was on the alert for something that would help it.

One day while I was talking with the parcel post man who delivered our parcel post to us, I found out that he also had arthritis. And he told me about a book called *Arthritis and Common Sense*—that he had used it, and that it had benefited him. I was intrigued by the title, so I sent to the publishers and got a copy. And when the book came, I was delighted with it. I find it to be everything that the title says. Just common sense, written in a language that anyone can understand.

I followed the directions given in the book faithfully, and within a month's time the swelling and the pain had gone from my hands. And now the daily pain-free use of my hands is a constant reminder of this grand little book, and what it did for me.

The above excerpts from the arthritis television program speak far more eloquently than I can. These are real people—typical victims of arthritis—telling their own story in their own way. Millions of TV viewers saw these people and heard this honest discussion.

Everywhere I travel, giving lectures, I am told how this conference-room scene in the TV film is convincing many Americans that my dietary theory is correct. The background facts on how the film was made and these quotes from the sound track have never been published before in a newspaper, magazine or book. They are so important to this issue of better health I have included them here for you to consider and discuss. You be the judge. Is diet effective against arthritis?

I am asking you to accept the idea that proper "lubrication" can relieve friction in "dried out" bodily joints. Once you agree to this basic theory, your next question will be about actual foods. What should you eat to gain adequate amounts of certain "oils"? The answer is a wide variety of appetizing foods—any of the items on the following list. . . .

FOODS RECOMMENDED FOR ARTHRITICS

MEATS

Beef, corned (very lean)	Kidney (beef)	Steak (sirloin, top round,
Chicken	Lamb chops (lean)	filet mignon, porterhouse,
Ham (lean)	Lamb, leg of (lean)	T-bone)
Hamburger (lean)	Liver	Tongue
Heart (beef)	Pork (center cut, lean)	Turkey
	Roast beef (lean)	Veal

FISH and SEAFOOD

Bluefish	Halibut	Scallops
Butterfish	Lobster	Shrimp
Clams	Mackerel	Swordfish
Codfish	Oysters	Tuna
Crab	Pompano	Trout
Flounder	Sardines	Whitefish
Haddock	Salmon	

VEGETABLES

Artichokes	Celery	Okra
Asparagus	Chard	Onions
Beans	Corn	Peas
Beets	Cucumber	Peppers
Beet greens	Dandelion greens	Potatoes
Broccoli	Eggplant	Radishes
Brussels sprouts	Endive	Spinach
Cabbage	Escarole	Squash
Carrots	Lettuce	String beans
Cauliflower	Lima beans	Tomatoes

FRUITS

Apples	Casaba melon	Pears
Apricots	Cherries	Plums
Bananas	Crenshaw melon	Prunes
Blackberries	Figs	Raisins
Blueberries	Honeydew melon	Raspberries
Cantaloupe	Peaches	Strawberries

When any of the above fruits come in canned form, be sure to drain away and discard the syrup. The sugar, concentrated in the syrup, is detrimental to arthritics.

DAIRY PRODUCTS

Cheeses	Eggs	Milk
American	Butter	(Homogenized vitamin-D
Blue		milk, pasteurized milk,
Cheddar		or raw milk, well shaken)
Cottage		
Cream		
Swiss		

BREADS

Bran or corn muffins	Cracked wheat bread	Rye
Brown bread	Graham or rye rolls	Whole wheat
Corn bread	Pumpernickel	

The above chart will give arthritics a "shopping list" to guide them during their next trip to a supermarket.

You will want to know how large a portion you should serve of these foods for various meals. For the proper quantities—and a daily selection of items to create a proper diet—consult the menus at the end of this chapter.

Perhaps you are surprised by the wide variety of tasty foods which are approved for arthritics. Yes, this dietary plan can be a pleasant experience. I am not proposing a "strict" diet, or asking you to starve yourself and exist on a set of strange foods.

In fact, you will find very few "health foods" or special products listed in the day-by-day menus. I have added some brewers' yeast, soya-lecithin granules, kelp and rose-hips powder (mostly with morning cereals) and some vitamin-mineral supplements. These are new elements which I have found to be beneficial to arthritics, based on new research since the publication of my previous book.

However, even with these additions, I'm sure you'll find that the menus are easy to follow, taste-appealing and more effective than ever! Remember, by depending on these foods, you will supply your body with the right types of dietary oils . . . to "lubricate" arthritic joints. To speed up this lubrication process, you must then turn to cod-liver oil.

For the Fastest Possible Relief—The Rules on Cod-Liver Oil

Throughout this book you have found repeated reference to the advantages of cod-liver oil as a dietary supplement. To gain maximum benefit, there is a definite way to take the oil. By combining oil with orange juice or milk, the entire mixture is more easily assimilated—it travels more readily from the stomach into the blood stream and reaches arthritic joints in greater supply.

Whenever you use cod-liver oil, whether for arthritis or as a dietary supplement to maintain good health, you should follow the procedure described below.

HOW TO MIX THE OIL AND JUICE

(You will need an orange, some cod-liver oil, a tablespoon, a juice strainer, and a small, screw-top jar.)

1. Take one half of a medium-size orange at room temperature. Squeeze out the juice and strain.
2. Put two tablespoons of strained orange juice into the jar. Make certain that all the pulp is removed.
3. Add one tablespoon of pure cod-liver oil to orange juice. (Use mint-flavored cod-liver oil, if you wish, for a more pleasant taste.) Cover and shake for 10 to 15 seconds. You will notice hundreds of tiny oil bubbles.
4. Drink the mixture immediately.
5. If the mixture is taken at night, do not disturb it by consuming food or water until at least four hours after taking the mixture. If the oil is taken in the morning, wait between one and two hours before eating or drinking. (The body will retain the organic iodine in the cod-liver oil more successfully if you follow this pre-eating and post-eating routine.)
6. Keep your bottle of cod-liver oil out of the sunlight. Keep it refrigerated at all times, to prevent it from becoming rancid.

7. It is important to use a small jar when mixing the ingredients. If you use a large jar, more of the oil will be left clinging to the inside surfaces of the jar—and your body will receive lesser amounts.

8. Do not mix the cod-liver oil with lemon or grapefruit juice. These juices are too acid. Orange juice or milk are the only liquids which should be used for mixing.

9. Do not use concentrated orange juice. It should be fresh and put through a strainer.

10. Do not use cod-liver oil capsules in place of bottled oil. The contents of capsules are quickly captured by the liver—cheating the linings of your joints, depriving them of lubrication.

11. After a certain period of time, you should start to taper down on the use of the cod-liver oil mixture. When? Cut down after you see that the dryness of hair and scalp has been corrected, when pain is relieved, when the normal supply of wax returns to your ears, when skin regains its luster. But do not stop the intake of cod-liver oil suddenly. Keep taking the mixture every other night, instead of daily. Continue this plan for approximately three months. Then use the oil at least twice each month.

12. Take cod-liver oil alone, without the orange juice if you wish. It has some advantages without the juice, particularly if you have arthritis in its advanced stages. (If you are deformed, for example, it would be wiser to mix the oil with two tablespoons of milk. Usually the deformed stage of arthritis indicates an allergy to the citric acid or fruit sugar in the orange.) After several months of oil and milk combinations—or straight oil—you may then use a small amount of the juice to mix the oil. For those who have not been ill too long—and are less sensitive to fruit juices—you can use up to four tablespoons of strained orange juice. But no one should use more than four tablespoons of juice with the oil.

The above rules on how to take the cod-liver oil mixture apply to millions of arthritics. They are effective in many types of arthritis, particularly for early and moderately advanced cases. I am the first to admit that no amount of cod-liver oil is going to reverse the crippling stage of arthritis. To anyone who already has frozen or disfigured joints, there is nothing other than possible surgery that can alter the condition. I do maintain, however, that proper diet and lubricating oils will check the advance of such cases and will reduce your pain. This is a blessing in itself.

The only exceptions to the 12 rules on mixing cod-liver oil are for people having other illnesses along with their arthritis. An arthritic who is also suffering from gall-bladder trouble, diabetes, high blood pressure or heart disease should mix the ingredients more thoroughly.

People with these ailments find that their bodies will not assimilate the oils quite so quickly, and therefore more mixing is required. They should take the cod-liver oil preparation only twice each week.

Arthritics with ulcers, dermatitis, psoriasis, eczema, skin irritations and nervous disorders, should take the cod-liver oil with milk or by itself (no orange juice).

Any arthritic who starts taking the mixture and then notices an accentuated pain in any of his joints may be experiencing some allergy. Merely stop using the orange juice—take the cod-liver oil with milk or straight.

Special Cod-Liver Oil Rules for Special Situations

For those who find the taking of the cod-liver oil mixture interferes with their daily schedule, we recommend the cod-liver oil mixture be taken over the week ends—on Saturdays and Sundays.

For those who find the cod-liver oil mixture difficult to take, we recommend the mixture be taken only twice a week, instead of daily.

For those who work late shifts or unusual hours, the cod-liver oil mixture can be taken to fit their working schedule and sleeping hours. It may be taken at whatever hour you arise, just as long as it is taken about one hour before the first meal and at least half an hour after any water intake. Or it can be taken just before going to sleep, at least four hours after any food intake. Or, if necessary, it can be taken just before leaving for work, providing it has been four hours since eating and at least one hour before any new food is to be taken.

All people without arthritis may take the cod-liver oil mixture as a preventive measure. Once a week is enough, after a two- to three-month period of daily intake. The one-time-a-week routine applies to those who have normal skin and no outward dryness. Generally a two- to three-month daily intake will correct any initial body dryness. The once-a-week routine is a maintenance program.

The above regimen applies to children as well as to adults.

If you are one of those who find that cod-liver oil "repeats," your system needs correction before you can take cod-liver oil. Add fat-splitting food supplements to your diet four or five times a week. Brewers' yeast and soya-lecithin granules are a must. Use one tablespoon of each on your cereal four or five times a week for at least six months. Then start using cod-liver oil twice a week, preferably only in the morning when the stomach is more likely to be empty. Skip breakfast on these two days a week. During the six months of no pure cod-liver oil, take a cod-liver oil emulsion like maltine daily before breakfast. It is much more palatable. It will be beneficial.

Those who cannot take the cod-liver oil mixture or an emulsion under any circumstances, should use the fat-splitting food supplements in their diet every other day, always. Follow the menus in this chapter with strict regularity. Depend more on correct diet plus brewers' yeast, soya-lecithin granules, rose-hips powder, kelp granules and high-quality vitamin and mineral products.

Is Cod-Liver Oil Fattening?

Some people hesitate when they hear about this cod-liver oil program. They fear that the plan will add inches to their waistline. You can relax and forget about this problem. One tablespoonful of cod-liver oil contains only 100 calories. And when the oil is taken on an empty stomach most of the oil is used for lubrication—not to produce energy or fat. You can retain your figure and normal weight levels.

Gout and Bursitis

Many who followed the arthritis diet for gout and bursitis have written to me of the relief obtained. Our clinical study gave added confirmation of our beliefs. This was also true in cases of neuritis and fibrositis, when these associated rheumatic problems occurred in patients studied.

Gout

Gout or gouty arthritis is a disorder in the uric acid metabolism of the body. Uric acid is a normal breakdown product of protein metabolism. We believe that if you assimilate your foods correctly no part of protein will cause any disturbance in the body.

The disorder in gout centers around the fluctuations of the uric acid content of the blood. Normally there are 2.5 to 5 milligrams of uric acid in every 100 cubic centimeters of blood in the blood stream, with an average of 3.5 milligrams. The blood of gouty persons contains abnormally high amounts.

If the uric acid content in the blood goes into the 6 to 8 milligram range, this is a forewarning of gout. One of three things is wrong:

1. The body is producing too much uric acid.
2. The kidneys cannot excrete uric acid fast enough.
3. The body cannot destroy excess uric acid.

If increased levels of uric acid persist, sodium urate crystals will eventually deposit in places like the big toe, cartilage, bursa, helix of the ear or in muscle tissue. Should these deposits go on for many years, these crystals will advance long enough to erode the tissue they invade and then may even replace the displaced portion.

Witching Hours and Ways

More often than not, gouty arthritis strikes during the sleeping hours. It attacks men almost 95 per cent of the time. It is believed that gout is inherited, but I do not subscribe to this belief.

Generally, the pattern is one of periodic episodes (lasting a few days to several weeks) of acute joint pain and swelling. Between attacks there may be almost complete remission, with restoration of normal joint function. As the disease goes into the chronic stages, it involves a number of joints, and tophaceous (chalky) deposits can frequently be found.

During the attacks, the sedimentation rate rises and the blood has an increased number of white blood cells trying to defend the body against the onslaught of pain. Fever and inflammation often accompany an attack, as do mild kidney changes.

Invariably the first attack involves the big toe, in-step, heel, ankle and knee. Initially, the big toe is ravaged 70 per cent of the time, then goes on to 90 per cent. Finally the legs become more and more susceptible to pain and swelling.

What About Diet and Gout?

Here is where I differ from the views set forth in medical literature. Gouty arthritics are often told to drink a lot of fluids. They are also told to avoid alcoholic beverages. The reason more of certain fluids are recommended is to avoid retention of concentrations of urates in the kidney tubules, which will lead to kidney damage.

I am for large amounts of liquid intake and against alcoholic beverages. But emphasis should be placed on the choice of liquids allowed with meals. All oil-free liquids should be kept away from foods in the process of digestion. Temperature of liquids should be considered. These factors are extremely vital to the program for recovery and prevention of future attacks. Above all, more stress to the liver must be avoided; otherwise the uric acid will be further disturbed.

I consider only three liquids should be allowed while the patient is recuperating. Room-temperature whole milk or warm soup (not fatty, not creamed) should be the only liquids allowed with meals.

Water, all you want, may be had but only at special

times. The kidneys should be literally flushed. The best time to drink water is upon arising, about one hour before breakfast, and again about half an hour before the evening meal, but at least five hours after lunch.

Avoid water after the evening meal. No iced liquids ever, especially none with or near meals. Don't congeal foods in your stomach, even temporarily. Forget beer and alcoholic beverages. It is also recommended that you give up coffee and tea.

Drinking oil-free liquids, especially after the large evening meal, is an invitation to further attacks. Taken this way, these liquids would increase the defects in digestion and assimilation. If this kind of mistake is continued, the need for colchicine could go on indefinitely.

The belief that particular purine foods, like sweetbreads, sardines and anchovies, cause gout is outdated.

Diet is important. A special consideration for the liquid part of the diet is a must. I think that gouty arthritics should look upon diet as their most important weapon. The menus in this chapter for arthritis are also recommended for victims of gout.

Bursitis

Bursitis is the inflammation of a single bursa, or many. There are a total of 140 bursae in the four extremities. Thirty-three bursae are in each arm; thirty-seven in each leg.

A bursa is a sac filled with a viscid fluid and situated at places in the tissues at which friction would otherwise develop. Bursae are lined with synovial membranes from which they take their nourishment, much like a joint lining. It is their small amount of fluid that allows movement between two surfaces.

Housemaid's knee, glass arm, musician's shoulder and tennis elbow are all popular expressions for some form of bursitis. The shoulder, however, seems to be bothered most often.

Bursitis in the Shoulder

Eighty per cent of all painful shoulders are due primarily to calcium deposits either in the subdeltoid muscle or its adjoining tendons.

A tendon is a fibrous cord of connective tissue in which the fibers of a muscle terminate and by which a muscle is attached to a bone or other structure.

Once these connective tissues start to wear out, they are highly susceptible to calcium deposits. Calcium-laden tendons can, as a result of a blow or injury, rupture and discharge calcium salts into the bursal sac. This release of calcium can offer temporary relief from a painful shoulder, but may go on to develop a calcium-filled bursa.

A painful shoulder seldom indicates arthritis. If no arthritis is evident but excruciating pain exists in the shoulder, more than likely the condition is bursitis.

Symptoms of acute subdeltoid bursitis include

tenderness or extreme shoulder pain on motion, possible radiation of the pain into the neck or down the arms. Blood tests, in acute attacks of bursitis, will show an increased sedimentation rate and an increased number of white blood cells, both of which indicate tissue inflammation.

What About Treatment?

The application of heat, temporary use of a sling and the use of aspirin is an acceptable pattern of early treatment.

Should pain persist, medical attention is required.

What About Diet and Bursitis?

In the matter of calcium deposits, sweets and sugar can be partially responsible. According to Dr. Melvin Page, who wrote *Degeneration-Regeneration,* an abundance of white sugar products in the diet upsets the calcium-phosphorus ratio in the blood. The phosphorus level goes down. Calcium goes up. This makes free calcium available, in unattached form. True, it may take many years of high sugar intake to undermine the body, but the results are devastating.

I say that calcium is best regulated by oil-soluble vitamin D, the kind found in cod-liver oil. Here is another reason to take <u>small amounts</u> of cod-liver oil <u>all your life</u>.

In addition, I am very much against anything that will literally starve the bursa's synovial membrane. Liquids that dry out the system actually starve the tissues. This means no soft drinks, juices, tea, alcoholic beverages or vinegar.

The menus recommended for bursitis are the same as for arthritis.

SEVEN DAYS OF MENUS FOR ARTHRITICS

FOR PEOPLE OF NORMAL WEIGHT

(SUGGESTED ALSO FOR VICTIMS OF GOUT AND BURSITIS)

MONDAY

BREAKFAST
Egg (soft-boiled). 3-minute
Rye toast .... 2 slices
Butter .... 1 pat
Cottage cheese ... ½ cup
Stewed prunes or black figs
Milk .... 8 oz.
Vitamin-mineral supplement
  (take with milk)

LUNCH
Choice of soup... 1 cup
Ry-krisp and butter
Apple .... large
Milk .... 10-oz. glass

DINNER
Vegetable soup ... 1 cup
Roast beef (lean). 6-8 oz.
Lettuce and tomato salad
Fruit in season
Milk .... 8 oz.

10 P.M.—11 P.M.

COD-LIVER OIL MIXTURE
  (Taken and mixed as described in
this chapter)

TUESDAY

BREAKFAST
Melon (in season) ½
Brown rice flake or bran and fig flake
  cereal:
Brewers' yeast
  (flake-form) ... 2 tbsp.
Soya-lecithin
  granules .... 1 tbsp.
Kelp granules .... ½ tsp.
Rose-hips powder . ½ tsp.
  (Mix four ingredients above into
last half-portion of cereal)
Milk .... 8 oz.

LUNCH
Graham or rye .... 1 roll
Butter .... 1 pat
Tossed green salad
  (choice of dressing, small amount)
Milk .... 8 oz.

DINNER
Chicken soup with
  brown rice...... 1 cup
Salmon steak
  (broiled) ...... 8 oz.
Baked potato .... medium
Sliced tomato .... 3 slices
Pear or apple
Milk .... 8 oz.

10 P.M.—11 P.M.
COD-LIVER OIL MIXTURE

WEDNESDAY

BREAKFAST

Oatmeal with milk 1 cup
"Raw" wheat germ 2 tbsp.
Brewers' yeast
  (flake-form) ... 2 tbsp.
Soya-lecithin
  granules .... 1 tbsp.
Kelp granules .... ½ tsp.
Rose-hips powder . ½ tsp.
  (Mix five ingredients above into
  last half-portion of cereal)
Choice of stewed prunes or melon in
  season
Milk .... 8 oz.

LUNCH

Chicken broth ... 1 cup
Broiled lean hamburger on roll
Sliced raw onion (optional)
Apple .... 1 large
Milk .... ½ glass

DINNER

Roast chicken ... ¼ (small)
Mashed potatoes.. ½ cup
Lima beans ...... ½ cup
Tomato and lettuce salad
Pear .... medium
Milk .... 8 oz.

10 P.M.—11 P.M.
COD-LIVER OIL MIXTURE

SPECIAL NOTE: In regard to drinking water, arthritics may have all they wish . . . just confine your drinking of water to twice a day. Upon arising—about one hour *before* breakfast— drink as much water as you desire. Additional water, any amount you wish, may be had at least one half hour before your evening meal.

THURSDAY

BREAKFAST

Poached eggs on toast
Cottage cheese ... ½ cup
Sliced banana and sour cream
Milk .... 8 oz.
Vitamin-mineral supplement
  (take with milk)

LUNCH

Minestrone soup.. 1 cup
Ry-krisp and butter
Fruit in season
Milk .... 8 oz.

DINNER

Oysters or clams on the half shell
Beef liver (broiled) 8 oz.
Steamed onions .. ¼ cup
Baked potato..... medium
Cantaloupe or melon in season
Milk .... 8 oz.

10 P.M.—11 P.M.
COD-LIVER OIL MIXTURE

FRIDAY

BREAKFAST

Rye bread
(buttered toast) 1 slice
Egg (poached) .. 1
Cottage cheese ... ½ cup
Choice of fruit
Milk .... 8 oz.
Vitamin-mineral tablet
(take with milk)

LUNCH

Choice of fish
Carrots (cooked). 3 or 4
Lima beans ...... ¼ cup
Milk .... 8 oz.

DINNER

Fish or meat course
Cole slaw
Baked potato..... medium
Celery sticks..... 2-3

10 P.M.—11 P.M.
COD-LIVER OIL MIXTURE

Several times a week, at the close of each breakfast, a vitamin-mineral tablet is suggested. Take this tablet *with whole milk* at the end of the meal. Use natural, organic vitamin-minerals. If available, use the *quick-dissolving* vitamin-mineral supplements.

SATURDAY

BREAKFAST

Brown rice flake cereal
Brewers' yeast
(flake-form) ... 2 tbsp.
Soya-lecithin
granules .... 1 tbsp.
Kelp granules .... ½ tsp.
Rose-hips powder. ½ tsp.
(Mix four ingredients above into
last half-portion of cereal)
Milk .... 8 oz.

LUNCH

Celery, watercress, tomato and escarole
salad and hard-boiled egg
Choice of dark
bread .... 1 slice
Butter .... 1 pat
Milk .... 8 oz.

DINNER

Choice of beef.... medium portion
Succotash .... ½ cup
String beans ..... ½ cup
Fruit salad ...... ½ cup
Milk .... 8 oz.

10 P.M.—11 P.M.
COD-LIVER OIL MIXTURE

SUNDAY

BREAKFAST

Choice of fruit in season
Corn or rye toast. 1 slice
Butter .... 1 pat
Canadian bacon or ham (lean)
Eggs (soft-boiled) 2
Milk .... 8 oz.
Vitamin-mineral tablet
  (take with milk)

DINNER

Lentil soup ...... 1 cup
Steak (broiled)... 8 oz.
Baked potato..... medium
Cabbage and raisin salad
Banana
Milk .... 8 oz.

SUPPER

Fruit salad (fresh) 1 cup
Sandwich (choice)
Crackers (wheat)
Milk .... 8 oz.

10 P.M.—11 P.M.
COD-LIVER OIL MIXTURE

The menus on these pages were designed for arthritics of normal weight. Space limitations of this volume prevent my listing complete menus for all weight groups. If you are underweight or overweight, and you have arthritis, may I suggest that you consult my earlier book, *Arthritis and Common Sense*. In that book, I list complete menus for people in each weight classification.

IMPORTANT REMINDER FOR ARTHRITICS
OF ALL WEIGHTS

THERE IS NO RULE WHICH SAYS THAT YOU MUST TAKE THE COD-LIVER OIL MIXTURE BETWEEN 10 P.M. AND 11 P.M. EACH NIGHT. YOU WILL NOTICE THAT THE 10 P.M. AND 11 P.M. HOURS WERE LISTED IN ALL OF THE MENUS ON THE PRECEDING PAGES. HOWEVER, THIS HOUR WAS GIVEN MERELY BECAUSE IT IS THE APPROXIMATE BEDTIME OF MANY ARTHRITICS.

THE POINT TO REMEMBER IS TO DRINK THE OIL MIXTURE AT LEAST FOUR HOURS AFTER YOUR EVENING MEAL. (WITH THE AVERAGE DINNER-TIME BEING ABOUT 6 P.M., THAT'S WHY THE 10 TO 11 P.M. HOUR MIGHT APPLY.) THEN, WHEN YOU RETIRE, THE OIL WILL REMAIN UNDISTURBED WHILE YOU SLEEP AND IT WILL HAVE A CHANCE TO BE ASSIMILATED. IF YOU PREFER, TAKE THE COD-LIVER OIL MIXTURE IN THE MORNING UPON ARISING . . . AT LEAST ONE HALF-HOUR AFTER YOU DRINK ANY WATER AND AT LEAST ONE HOUR BEFORE EATING BREAKFAST.

Chapter XIV

Strictly Personal: Answers from the Author

Any thinking person, when he hears about a new theory or reads about new ideas, will want to ask questions. Before you accept the opinions of an author, you have every right to inquire about his qualifications. Does he have the personal experience, the knowledge and the background to deserve your support? Does he <u>know</u> what he's talking about?

I welcome the opportunity to discuss my past history, to give you a brief "autobiography," so you can judge for yourself whether I have had the proper preparation to write on the subject of diet and nutrition.

Some readers might think it immodest of me, might wonder why I am including autobiographical facts in this book. It is not ego, believe me. On the contrary, I shall now tell you about my critics, my detractors, and how I became a "controversial figure" in the medical world.

I have always believed that the public is entitled to complete information about an author and his work. When my previous book on arthritis became a topic of national interest, *Life* magazine decided to do an article and picture layout about me. I cooperated fully with their writers and research staff. *Life* did an excellent job of reporting the story; they covered both the negative and positive factors and they published seven pages of impartial truth.

As part of my desire to tell all the facts, I then accepted an invitation to answer the most probing questions in television. I appeared on the famous "Nightbeat" program—where Mike Wallace cross-examined, dissected and challenged his guests. A huge audience of TV viewers saw Mike Wallace put me under the "Nightbeat" microscope.

It had taken many years of work, research, study and personal contact with thousands of arthritics before national magazines and network television shows saw fit to discuss my book and my theories on nutrition.

My book was first published in 1951. By 1953, public demand had caused *Arthritis and Common Sense* to have nine printings and three editions. But the turning point had not yet been reached . . . the most dramatic events were still ahead.

One incident would now change the entire course of my life. The hero—or villain—would be television. I already knew the power of TV, the fact that it reached into millions of homes. My half-hour television film (the panel discussion with Conrad Nagel, described previously) was already being seen in scores of cities. But I was completely unprepared for the fantastic results of the Arthur Godfrey program.

It began quietly enough one morning when Peter Lind Hayes was substituting for Mr. Godfrey and was

chatting casually with his TV viewers. Mrs. Grace Hayes
—Peter's mother—had written him a letter from her
home in Nevada. For years she had been a victim of
arthritis. Peter told his listeners how his mother had
suddenly reported an improvement in her health.

A friend of hers had recommended my book, Mrs.
Hayes had read it, and within a few weeks she was feeling very much better. In her case my dietary plan worked
where other methods had failed.

Peter Lind Hayes mentioned her experience merely
as an item of possible interest to other arthritics. Little
did he know the nationwide reaction his comments would
cause.

Within 48 hours, the mail began to pour in. Letters came from other arthritics praising my book, reporting that they too had been helped through proper
diet. Peter showed some of these letters on camera and
discussed them on the air. Interest was so great that
arrangements were then made to have me come to New
York. I appeared on the program, was interviewed and
answered questions about the book.

Almost overnight the whole country wanted to read
my suggestions on diet. More than 25,000 copies of the
book were sold in a matter of days. *The New York Times*
and the *New York Herald Tribune* began to show the
title on their best-seller lists.

If the story ended here—on a high note of success
—it could be compared to Horatio Alger. But this happy
picture was due to change to a personal nightmare. I

would soon have to face a series of shocking developments.

Every author has his share of critics. And I certainly didn't expect everyone to agree with my views on nutrition. Constructive criticism is always welcome. But an outright attack—on your personal reputation, your motives, your freedom to write and be heard—is hard to take calmly. I find myself in a battle, and I intend to fight back!

Because of *Arthritis and Common Sense* I have been criticized, cross-examined and even denounced. It is time, now, that I answer and tell my side of this great debate.

The controversy began—it swung into high gear—soon after the Arthur Godfrey television program. Until that time the medical profession apparently considered me just a minor annoyance. However, when my book climbed the best-seller lists to the number-one spot, someone must have decided it was time to challenge Alexander. Perhaps too many people were beginning to follow my dietary plan, or too many people were starting to achieve results!

The assertion that a person could "do something about arthritis, right in his own home" was enough to make some doctors antagonistic, even though I emphasized that readers should consult their physicians regularly for examinations, progress reports, etc. While I favor certain forms of home remedy, I am not antidoctor, not antimedicine.

Next, my critics released a flood of negative publicity centering around the fact that my dietary regimen "had not been clinically tested." The implication was that my diet was not worth testing—or that I was avoiding such a clinical evaluation.

The true facts are that I had aggressively sought a formal test—in a recognized clinic or hospital—for more than five years. Among the institutions I approached were the Arthritis and Rheumatism Foundation, the National Institute of Public Health, the New York Hospital for Joint Diseases . . . urging them to try my dietary program among arthritic patients. All these organizations declined.

Through congressmen in Washington, I tried time and again to have governmental health agencies conduct clinical tests. I offered to donate royalties from my book to underwrite the entire cost of a scientific analysis—to prove or disprove my theories.

Finally, in 1957, a clinic in Massachusetts did conduct an evaluation among actual patients. The very favorable results are described in Chapter XXI.

The arguments against my nutritional program for arthritics included some amazing errors on the part of my critics. For instance, they often implied that the readers of my book were merely gaining "psychosomatic" relief . . . that it was all "mental." This comment may seem rather nonsensical to the 700,000 Americans who now own copies.

Another tactic by the opposition was to claim that

my book was only a means of "temporary" relief. Or, rather, that the book was not responsible for any relief . . . the patient was simply experiencing "a temporary regression, a normal easing of pain and symptoms." In reply, I can cite case histories where the reader has enjoyed eight years of continuing good health.

I have no quarrel with anyone who wants to debate legitimate questions about nutrition, diet, menus, etc. But I strongly object when the issue is sidetracked and the critics assail a man's personal reputation. In order to discredit the book, there was a campaign to deprecate and denounce the author.

My lack of formal education was made the primary target during the controversy. I did not have a medical degree; therefore how could I understand anything about arthritis? How dare I write a book on a health subject? "After all, he's just a layman!"

Organized medicine issued many statements deploring my "lack of qualifications." They ignore the fact that I have now spent fifteen years studying arthritis, talking in person with actual victims of the illness. Through my lectures—always followed by question-and-answer sessions—I have met more arthritics than any man alive today. And my book today reflects not only my own experience, but also all that I have learned from contact with 300,000 arthritics.

Because of my writings and my constant lecture tours, I have been accused of having a fanatic interest in my work. "He's on a personal crusade to conquer arthritis!" True. But is that a motive to be condemned?

According to my critics, sincerity is a vice and "laymen" are ignorant.

"But truth prevails. ARTHRITIS AND COMMON SENSE continues to grow in popularity. It is now in its 38th printing since published 23 years ago. Sales, all in hard cover, have surpassed the 925,000 mark. The book has been Anglicized in Great Britain for the British Empire. It has been translated into German, Spanish, and more recently into the Danish language. It is expected to be translated into Japanese, French, and Italian in the near future.

Doctors who now write their own books on ARTHRITIS constantly refer to the cod liver oil regime and unique eating habits expressed by Dale Alexander's revolutionary book ARTHRITIS AND COMMON SENSE. Alexander's book on Arthritis was the first book published of its kind in the world relating the problem of arthritis to poor nutrition and improper eating habits.

The Los Angeles Times in 1973 listed ARTHRITIS AND COMMON SENSE as one of the top 100 books written in the last century. It was placed alongside of such other notable books as POWER OF POSITIVE THINKING (Dr. Norman Vincent Peale), FANNIE FARMER'S COOKBOOK . . . and Dr. Spock's book on Baby Care.

I hope that the past few pages have given you a clear view of the controversy. I have talked with you frankly and openly . . . so you will know both sides of this debate.

There will be more newspaper headlines, television interviews, pro and con discussions. I have no doubt that the publication of this book will launch another phase of this remarkable story. The ending is not yet known. In fact, as you read this book today, you become part of the entire picture . . . and you are helping to write the final chapters.

Will public opinion support these new ideas on nutrition . . . cause the medical world to accept diet as the key weapon??? Will COMMON SENSE prevail???

Chapter XV

High Blood Pressure, Poor Circulation, Hardening of the Arteries, Gall-Bladder Ailments

If your blood pressure is high, you are told to lose weight. The chances are good that when you lose 15 to 20 pounds, your blood pressure will go down. However, more ·often than not, it is a temporary reduction.

Every time you gain weight, blood pressure fluctuates between normal and abnormal. This is a serious situation. This problem is generally accompanied by the closely related disorders of poor blood circulation and hardening of the arteries. The three ailments frequently are interwoven. If you have one, you have the makings of all three.

Moderate weight gain and weight reduction can take place without affecting the body. But it requires knowing how to eat properly so that selected foods are adequately assimilated. Eventually, though, too much weight gain will upset the scales of better health.

Many people are in the throes of gaining or losing 15 to 20 pounds several times a year, most of their lives. They put it on, then take it off, and during a span of ten years or so, perhaps 300 to 400 pounds are exchanged. As a rule, this leads to permanent high blood pressure, impaired blood circulation and eventually the inevitable hardening of the arteries. These problems are closely associated with blood cholesterol disturbance. Heart disease is not too far away.

On the other hand, these disorders may occur without any weight change. Proper assimilation of foods can do much to deter circulatory disorders.

The body cannot live on an oil-free diet. If you are already faced with problems like high blood pressure, poor blood circulation, hardening of the arteries, high blood serum cholesterol and heart disease, you should be on a low-fat diet. But this diet must contain moderate amounts of the vital oils like those found in milk, eggs and limited amounts of cod-liver oil (see Chapter VI). Otherwise your body will go one way—downhill— through a process of slow degeneration accompanied by all the problems associated with old age.

Poor Circulation

Circulatory disorders are preceded by a variety of danger signals—occasional spasms in an extremity, increasing attacks of prickly tingling in an arm or leg, frequent periods of a limb falling asleep and finally the dread realization of actual numbness. Also, as you grow older you realize that your hands and feet seem to be getting colder.

In my opinion, impaired blood circulation is the first step toward high blood pressure and hardening of the arteries. All three diseases are tied to the problem of blood-sludging.

The constant intake of inferior oil-bearing foods—like bacon fat, oleomargarine with its basic lack of iodine, potato chips, French fries, peanuts roasted in overheated oil, fried doughnuts and many similar foods—floods the system. The body can handle so much of these inferior oils; then it will begin to rebel and develop disorders.

Drinking oil-free liquids with oily foods will start the blood-sludging problem. The colder the liquid, the faster the pace of trouble develops. To avoid poor circulation of blood, I believe it will be advisable to follow the menus in Chapter VI.

High Blood Pressure

We speak of blood pressure in numerical terms expressed in millimeters. A blood pressure reading is believed to be normal when it is in the 120-millimeter range. A blood pressure measurement can be obtained on a special apparatus known as a sphygmomanometer. When the heart is resting between its pumping efforts, a reading of 80 millimeters is considered normal. Most of us are concerned when more than 120 millimeters of pressure are required by our heart muscle to pump blood throughout our system. Some 15 million Americans suffer from some degree of high blood pressure.

The same mistakes that cause poor circulation of

the blood, I believe, go on to cause high blood pressure. Also, but in a secondary role, kidney, nervous system and glandular disease can raise blood pressure. The modern trend of eating highly salted foods is throwing an overload on the kidneys.

These foods make the kidneys work harder. They cause a constricting effect on blood vessels in the kidneys. This means the heart too must work harder.

Rats placed on high salt diets have had their blood pressure raised. There is much medical literature recommending salt-free diets in the treatment of high blood pressure.

Dr. Frederick J. Stare, professor of nutrition at Harvard, believes that excess salt may be hurting more Americans than even saturated fats. He points out that adults normally need only about half a gram of salt a day. I estimate, however, that most people consume 10-15 grams, and much of it is already incorporated in the food they buy.

The human heart, as a pump, adjusts itself to the various conditions to which it is subjected. Stress, emotional disturbances, fright, violent exercise all can cause the heart to pound faster. Prolonged physical work speeds up the pumping of blood. The blood pressure rises, but this kind of rise is generally temporary.

A visit to a doctor can raise the blood pressure. This kind of hypertension is, more often than not, adequately stabilized by the endocrine gland system and is not a disease.

But the kind of blood pressure that remains high is extremely hard on the glands. Something is wrong. Drugs will not correct the underlying disorder. True, the heart-pumping action is slowed down by drugs, but the fault is still going to remain antagonistic to the blood pressure level. Stop the drugs and the pressure goes up again. During our clinical study on arthritis, no blood pressure medication or drugs were used. Yet with correct diet and eating habits, we noted impressive changes for the better.

We noted a consistent pattern of reduction in blood pressure findings, when abnormally high levels existed at the beginning of the study:

CASE 37: Male, 62 years old.

DATE	BLOOD PRESSURE	WEIGHT
7/23/57	160/95	192
9/2/57	140/75	186
11/23/57	124/70	188½

CASE 68: Male, 39 years old.

DATE	BLOOD PRESSURE	WEIGHT
7/24/57	150/90	181
11/29/57	130/88	175½

CASE 1: Female, 61 years old.

DATE	BLOOD PRESSURE	WEIGHT
7/18/57	190/80	131
11/21/57	144/90	126½

Weight change varied very little, relatively speaking. Furthermore, the patients were taking whole milk, eggs, butter and cod-liver oil. They were simply taught how to eat so that what they ate would be absorbed in a way beneficial to their bodies.

Hardening of the Arteries

Usually, when poor circulation of the blood and high blood pressure persist, the arteries are getting increasingly hardened. Properly selected oils in your food should be helping to keep the arteries elastic.

Poor eating habits have the opposite effect. Body oils that should be soluble become insoluble. Calcium, instead of helping the body, plays a role in the process of hardening the fatty deposits in the arteries. The entire physiology of the body is unbalanced.

Several supplemental foods could help keep oils more soluble and on the move. One such important food is soybean-lecithin granules.

The medical doctor who established the value of soybean-lecithin granules in relief of cholesterol and hardening of the arteries is Dr. Lester M. Morrison, author of *The Low-Fat Way to Health and Longer Life*. His dietary program has been shown to be an effective method of preventing and treating hardening of the arteries. His concentrates of de-fatted soya-lecithin were found to lower blood serum cholesterol. Lecithin is now acknowledged as a fat-emulsifier.

I highly approve of using soya-lecithin granules daily if you have had a history of heart disease, high blood pressure or impaired blood circulation. I highly recommend that everyone use soya-lecithin granules several times a week, even if nothing seems to be wrong. It rides hard on fat disorders before they can occur. Soya-lecithin granules contain ingredients that cod-liver oil lacks: the fat-dispersing properties of choline and inositol, vitamins of the B-complex.

Dr. Morrison is also in favor of brewers' yeast and wheat germ. In his book he claims that his dietary regimen was capable of internally dissolving the fatty, yellowish plaques over the eyes and in the skin wherever found. These are often seen in people with circulatory disorders.

If, however, you insist on drinking oil-free liquids with foods that contain oils, I say you are also unnecessarily taxing an important organ, the gall bladder. Let's spend a few minutes together learning something about gall bladders and gallstones. It will add to our knowledge.

The Gall Bladder and Correct Eating Habits

The gall bladder is a storage tank for bile. Made by the liver, the bile flows through the biliary duct down past the gall bladder and into the intestine. There it aids in the digestion and absorption of the fatty foods you eat.

When there is no fat to be digested the opening through which liver bile goes into the intestine closes itself. This detours the bile into the gall bladder, where it is retained until needed. Sometimes, by processes not clearly understood, elements of this bile may crystallize to form a hard little mass called a stone. As time goes on the stone may become larger as more crystallized bile

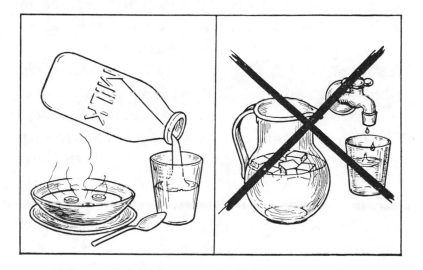

Drink ONLY room-tempera-
ture milk or warm soup
with your meals.

NEVER drink water with
meals, or iced water at any
time.

forms around it, or additional stones may be formed. These stones can cause trouble by blocking the passage out of the gall bladder and/or by irritating the bladder.

The kinds of people who are susceptible to gall-bladder disease are obese individuals, diabetics, those recuperating from heart attacks, and others with poorly functioning thyroids.

One out of five adults eventually gets gall-bladder disease. Half of all women in their sixties have gall-bladder problems. They go to surgery eight times more frequently than men.

Can correct diet and eating habits help you to avoid or reduce the chances of gall-bladder trouble? Yes, to a considerable extent. It seems clear that gall-bladder trouble is a matter of faulty digestion or absorption of fats. Therefore you should exercise care as to how and when you consume fats, and as to which fats to avoid.

I have outlined here a little guide to help you, but I want to emphasize that it is very important to keep away from iced liquids with or near fatty meals. Your gall bladder may react with spasms at first and severe pain later on. I believe iced beverages and oil-free liquids in conflict with oily foods going through the process of digestion are long-range diet mistakes that will cause gall-bladder attacks eventually if not immediately.

SENSIBLE RULES AND EATING HABITS

1. Avoid iced liquids with or near foods that contain oil.
2. Avoid oil-free liquids with meals. (This means no coffee or tea.)
3. Do not go on an oil-free diet. If you do, you may help your gall bladder but you will also dry out your skin, joints, eyes, ears and entire body. It is not a fair exchange.
4. You may go on a low-fat diet. But whole milk, some eggs (soft-boiled) and limited amounts of cod-liver oil must be left in the diet.
5. A cod-liver oil mixture, about twice a month, should be

taken in place of breakfast, when the stomach is completely empty. (See Chapter XIII.)

6. Soya-lecithin granules, as a food supplement, should be added to the diet. Use one tablespoonful on your cereal or on soup, three or four times a week. Lecithin of this kind will do the most good to keep the fats in your blood stream emulsified. If you have trouble handling fats, soya-lecithin granules are a must. Use small amounts indefinitely.

7. Skim milk with meals is not the answer to gall-bladder attacks.

8. The best menus we could recommend for those with gall-bladder problems are the menus in Chapter VI which are suggested for the prevention of heart disease.

9. Learn to drink water as advised throughout this book. It is most important that you do, especially if you take any pills or tablets of any description, be they medication or vitamin supplements.

Chapter XVI

Dry Skin, Acne and Other Skin Problems
—And Your Diet

If your skin is normal, ordinarily you do not give it too much thought. Most people, beyond the childhood years, do not have healthy skin. It may appear healthy and supposedly normal, but closer inspection raises doubt.

Look for: tendency to dryness, oily areas, enlarged or prominent skin pores, scattered areas of blackheads, pus pimples, boils, inclination to wrinkles, loss of skin tone, overgrowth of facial hair, surface plaques or cholesterol around the eyes, eczema, scurf and scaliness, receding hairline, dandruff—these are but a few of the warnings that the skin is in trouble.

In this chapter, we will consider some of the more common problems of skin disease.

Dry Skin

For the past fifteen years I have written and lectured on the belief that dry skin is chiefly caused by soft drinks, tea, frozen and fresh fruit juices, excessive amounts of the more caustic citric fruits, mixed drinks with soda, seltzer and Vichy and the use of vinegar.

Our clinical findings substantiated these beliefs. Sixty-eight per cent of the patients exhibited some degree of dry skin, scalp and hair. Simultaneously, brittle fingernails (part of the skin) were a frequent occurrence.

Admittedly we do not know just how the aforementioned foods operate to dry out the skin. From observation and persistent study, however, we do know that they were used excessively. Sometimes it was found that their prolonged use was not a current dietary mistake. But closer scrutiny of past dietary habits generally located a time when these foods played a major role in their diet.

When these acid-type foods—beverages particularly—were completely eliminated, the skin problems of our arthritic patients responded favorably. In my opinion, the body had been giving up its neutralizing or buffer salts in its effort to keep the blood from getting acid.

These neutralizing substances are borrowed from the skin earlier than from any other organ. If acid and caustic-type foods and beverages are continued in the diet, the health of most organs will eventually be sacrificed, organ by organ. The skin is generally the first to be adversely affected by wrong foods. This is an accepted fact in medical literature on skin diseases. By the same token, I believe the skin can be reconditioned first by a correct diet.

Often, as literature points out, medical science is slow to find the exact explanation for conditions whose causes are common knowledge. It is only a matter of time before alert scientists will give us the explanation of dry skin in terms of biochemical changes responsible for the phenomena.

The Oily-Skin Problem

We observed in our study that patients using oleomargarine in place of butter often had oily foreheads and faces. Some complained of literally oiling their pillow-cases during a night's sleep.

Substantiation of skin sensitivity to the kind of fatty acids found in oleomargarine can be found in medical textbooks. Such evidence exists in the book *Modern Nutrition in Health and Disease* by Wohl and Goodhart. In the chapter "Absorption, Digestion and Metabolism of Fats," Dr. H. J. Deuel, Jr., professor of biochemistry and nutrition at the University of Southern California, notes that linoleic types of fatty acids cause extraordinary skin sensitivity.

I note that oleomargarine contains large amounts of linoleic fatty acids. Recently there has been a growing race between manufacturers of this product to increase its content of these particular fatty acids for "heart customers."

Regardless of who uses oleomargarine, an excessive amount of this kind of product for a number of months or years will overpower the sebaceous glands. These oil glands can hold only so much and when they overspill, the fatty secretion (sebum) is discharged to the skin surfaces. It flows out from the glands through the spaces between the walls of the hair follicles and into the small openings of the skin.

Chemically, this oily film consists of fatty acids (whatever is in the food you are eating), cholesterol and other fatty derivatives.

We find that most people who eat a great deal of potato chips, roasted peanuts, fatty bacon, sausages and their like, meat fats, cold cuts, hydrogenated peanut butter and certain salad oils have oil film covering their skin and scalp.

Acne

We believe these layers of oil film increase the vulnerability to acne. This is an ailment marked by the presence of pimply swellings called acne lesions.

The full cause of acne is unknown, at least according to the dermatologists, medical textbooks and articles on the subject. I would like to offer my interpretation of its development:

1. Wrong oils in the diet are dispersed almost uniformly throughout all fat deposits of the body. The areas of the skin over the forehead, nose, face, chest and trunk contain the greatest number of oil glands.
2. An abundance of inferior diet oils will fill these oil glands to overflowing capacity. At this point, further dietary increase will cause an overflow into the skin.

3. More often than not, these oils are of the saturated variety. These are classified as insoluble types.

4. Once these insoluble grades of oils are discharged into the oil-gland ducts, they are not easily burned off (oxidized) as energy. Continuous secretions of sebum begin to block the duct-shafts leading to the outer skin. This failure to be oxidized or used up may be the point at which blackheads begin to form. Acne lesions may soon develop.

Other factors may enter into the reason for blackhead formation. The Drs. Sutton, in their book *Diseases of the Skin,* believe that fats predispose to the development of blackheads. They are against inferior oils like those in ice cream and chocolate, favorite foods of the young.

Acne appears most frequently in teen-agers. The adolescent years parallel peculiar (even if temporary) eating habits. Most youngsters eat an enormous amount of sweets.

In searching for the cause of acne, medical researchers point out that high carbohydrate diets increase the susceptibility and effects of infection. Drs. Wise and Sulzberger, well-known dermatologists, note that the "ill effects of a relatively high carbohydrate intake of sweets and starches may not be due so much to the actual high carbohydrate intake but rather to an idiosyncrasy in reaction toward certain specific items in the carbohydrate diet." They specifically mention foods like chocolate and white bread.

Throughout the literature on skin diseases, dermatologists agree that chocolate increases the vulnerability to acne. Others also indict pastries, malted-milk shakes, candy, pie, cake, sherbet and refined gelatin products. If acne lesions are present, it is believed sweets will spread the inflammation.

Not only do adolescents overindulge in sweets, but also in fried foods. Once any oil is subjected to high heat, it has no value to the skin or tissue. Furthermore, superheated oils, whether they are high- or low-quality oils, are antagonistic to the repair of the skin.

Many popular items among teen-agers—potato chips, French fries, popcorn, pretzels, crackers, peanuts, etc.—are oversalted. In no time at all, a huge amount of salt can enter the blood stream, putting a tremendous strain on the kidneys.

In addition, much of this salt is oxidized. This inorganic type of iodine could stimulate the thyroid to speed up the body metabolism. This would mean bursts of energy, with worse rebounds. Meanwhile, the temporary bursts of increased metabolism probably cause the oil glands to discharge more of the wrong oils.

What is needed to get children through their adolescence and periods of fast growth rate is the organic iodine in oils like cod-liver oil, not inorganic iodine. Correct choices of iodized foods and oils will be of immense value to the glands, hormonal system and growth.

I want to make it clear that wrong foods are not the sole cause of acne, but in my opinion they are frequently

responsible for triggering acne, and I believe that overheated food oils and huge amounts of salt cause far
more trouble than sweets. Together, these particular
foods open the door to greater skin sensitivity.

Once this sensitivity exists in the skin, allergies
can multiply tenfold. Even beneficial sugars, if highly
concentrated like those in apricots, figs, prunes and
dates, will now cause the skin to flare up, especially if
there is an accompanying vitamin-B deficiency. Normally, this would not occur.

Other than correcting your eating habits, rely on
warm water and mild soap for keeping the skin clean as
well as clear. Keep away from face powder, pancake
bases and skin lotions. These will clog the pores. And
remember: you cannot wash faulty diet off your skin.

Psoriasis

Here is the most common skin disease seen in the
skin clinics. Nearly one million people in the United
States have psoriasis in some degree. The first outbreak
is usually a flat, red area which later becomes covered
with silvery scales. This may spread and join with others
to form larger areas. Common sites are the elbows,
knees, arms, lower back and scalp.

Our experience indicates that frozen and fresh
juices (especially grapefruit and lemon), soft drinks,
Vichy, seltzer, the combination of tea and lemon, an
abundance of white sugar and vinegar are the special

foods which lead skin-sensitivity problems into the area
of psoriasis.

Psoriatic arthritics responded to our dietary regimen. Scientific literature indicates psoriatic skins need
specific fatty acid replacement. Tablets of undecylenic
acid are prescribed by some dermatologists.

Dr. William Brady's syndicated newspaper column
indicates that people following his iodine ration find
relief for their psoriasis. Remember the cod-liver oil
used in our dietary regimen contains iodine.

Often psoriatic conditions in pregnant women will
clear up automatically. On the other hand, emotional
stress will worsen psoriasis for them. The blood of a
pregnant woman is rich in iodine. Emotional disturbances upset the pituitary, a natural reservoir of iodine.

Eczema

In England, the successful choice of treatment for
eczema is the use of cod-liver oil. In our country, various
other remedies have been tried, with indifferent results.

Oils That Help Your Skin Need Help from
Other Vitamins

If you take cod-liver oil in mixture form (see Chapter XIII) for its valuable fatty acids, the essential oils
it contains work best when other vitamins are simultaneously available in the diet.

Dr. H. E. Worne, in *Archives of Research* (August,

1954), says the pyridoxine part of the vitamin-B complex and vitamin C are both important for one to gain maximum benefits from fatty acids.

Dr. Louis Tulipan of New York uses brewers' yeast in treating acne in older people. He observed 96 patients over a period of eight years, prescribed a diet rich in vitamins and supplemented with brewers' yeast.

Dr. H. Lawrence, well-known dermatologist and author of *The Care of Your Skin,* suggests that readers of his book ask their doctors to suggest a multivitamin preparation to be taken with each meal.

Skin Education Program for Teen-Agers and Everyone

The vital years of adolescence are crucial to the lifetime beauty of the skin. We believe special educational material should be available in schools regarding food and beverages and their relationship to skin problems. Meanwhile, we offer the following guide:

Grades of Oil-Bearing Foods

GOOD: Milk, eggs, butter and cod-liver oil.
BAD: Bacon fat, oleomargarine, oils used in preparation of potato chips, roasted peanuts, French fries, doughnuts, hydrogenated peanut butter, pastries, chocolate, candy, ice cream, etc.

Grades of Carbohydrates (Starches and Sweets)

GOOD: Whole-grain breads and cereals, baked potatoes.
BAD: Devitalized white bread, refined macaroni, spaghetti, refined cereals, etc.

Grades of Sweets

GOOD: Natural sugars as found in fresh and dried fruits and in vegetables.

BAD: White sugar, candy, pie, cakes, cookies, soft drinks, ice cream, sherbet, refined gelatin desserts, etc.

Grades of Salt

GOOD: That which exists as natural mineral salts in fresh fruit and vegetables.

BAD: Excessive table salt. Especially bad is the "treated" salt used on roasted peanuts, potato chips, etc.

Grades of Protein Foods

GOOD: Dairy products, lean meats, brewers' yeast.

BAD: Sausages and cold cuts mixed with chemicals, pre-packaged protein foods that have been refined or preserved.

To maintain a normal skin, fresh fruits and vegetables, lean meats and dairy products are not enough. The term "dairy products," for instance, is too vague. One needs to include whole milk in the selection of dairy products to have a radiant, alive-looking skin.

Chapter XVII

Ulcers and Colitis

The story about "my ulcer" may sound familiar to some of you.

It took shape during my service in the Air Force in World War II. I was assigned to the Station General Hospital in San Antonio and was a laboratory helper at that hospital.

The food was good, as military fare goes, and access to the hospital kitchen was easy. At this time I developed a liking for pineapple juice, and within a few weeks I consumed many, many cans of this liquid.

Then it happened: severe pains just above the pit of my stomach that would last up to a half hour. They seemed like hunger pains. My stools became tarry.

According to medical literature, tarry stools could indicate an ulcer. Textbooks said gastric-ulcer pain came thirty to sixty minutes after meals. My pain, coming three or four hours after eating, seemed to fit the description of a duodenal ulcer. Some books lumped the two types together under the broader term of peptic ulcer and stated that duodenal ulcers were the more common.

Generally, in the diagnosis for a stomach ulcer a specimen of gastric juice is removed from the stomach

by way of a tube passed down through the mouth. From
this sample, it is determined how much free and total
hydrochloric acid is present under fasting conditions.
This is then compared to a test meal. Abnormally high
amounts of this stomach acid are usually found in ulcer
victims.

Direct examination with a fluoroscope or X-ray
photography, following a barium test meal, can also be
used for diagnostic purposes. The ulcer crater, if present, can be seen in X-ray pictures.

When the stomach is empty, pain is generally experienced by the ulcer patient. It is due to the highly
acid stomach juices on the open wound when no food
(like milk) is present to dilute the gastric juice.

Constant stretching and relaxing of the stomach
and continual activity of digestion in the duodenum can
also affect the healing process. Recurrence after healing
is frequent.

In my case, because of my close observation of
food intake during my studies on arthritis before coming
into the service, I could immediately pinpoint the one
new food in my diet: pineapple juice. This was stopped
and I started to drink quarts of milk.

The change in stool color cleared up in about three
days and the customary pain after meals gradually sub-
sided.

My experience is not held out to mean that everyone who drinks excessive amounts of pineapple juice
will get an ulcer. It is only part of my story.

Ulcers, Onions and Spices

About a year later, I decided to introduce another new food to my diet. My wife and I were sharing an apartment in New York City with another couple, and I noticed he ate a great deal of onions. I was struck by his healthy-looking crop of hair and wondered if my thinning hair might benefit by some raw onion. Up to then, my twenty-ninth year, I had never eaten raw onion. However, I soon found that too much of this raw vegetable caused "repeating."

About two years later, I decided to try onion again, but this time mixed into an omelet. For six months, two or three times a week, that was my breakfast, with a whole medium-size onion in each preparation. When the sharp epigastric pain returned, I gave up onion. It had been helpful in two ways: checking the rapid hair loss and being instrumental in better bowel regularity.

Over the course of the next few years, I was compelled to give up all mustard, black pepper, relishes, spices, chives, scallions, garlic, and fresh pineapple. Still, I do not say that any of these foods used individually and in moderation will necessarily cause an ulcer. On the contrary, they are excellent contributions to anyone's diet. But taken excessively, they may well take part in the development of an ulcer.

Textbooks, Medical Journals and Ulcers

In medical journals and textbooks, the opinions seem to be that an ulcer is an eroded lesion in the mucous membrane that resists healing. In Chapter VII we looked upon cancer as a frustrated attempt by the body to heal a wound; an ulcer can become cancerous. It has the disadvantage of being subjected constantly to acid gastric juices. Milk and cream can do much to control hydrochloric acid for hours at a time.

Textbooks also indicate that people with ulcers also have low vitamin C levels. Without normal amounts of this vitamin, ulcers will not heal well. My trouble was caused apparently by a fruit juice rich in vitamin C, too much, too soon.

As a child, I did not have much fresh orange juice. It was a luxury item in the family budget. Instead, we had an abundance of overripe bananas, for the price of ten cents a dozen.

At the age of twelve I began to drink extremely large amounts of carbonated drinks. While attending the movies, sometimes as much as three times a week, I had more than my share of candy bars and potato chips. A purchase of rich pastry became a daily habit after I delivered the morning newspapers on my route. Another favorite was cold-cut sandwiches with huge amounts of mustard. This certainly was not beneficial.

As a teen-ager I had no ulcer-type pain at all. But

with the consumption of all that corrosive mustard and the erosive action of the enormous amounts of carbonated drinks, it is possible that a great deal of vitamin C was needed by my body to keep the stomach membrane repaired. I always drank a good deal of milk.

By the time I reached the Air Force, the long years of improper food punishment probably put me in a highly susceptible position for an ulcer. The sudden intake of excessive amounts of pineapple juice most likely was the *coup de grâce*. But the earlier mistakes had set the stage.

Look at the carbonated drink, candy and pastry part of my diet and then consider what Dr. D. T. Quigley says about ulcers, in an article published in the *Nebraska State Journal* (April, 1945):

> . . . peptic ulcer is a deficiency disease reflecting a relatively high intake of refined carbohydrates and an inadequate amount of all vitamin and food minerals. A high vitamin and mineral diet should be prescribed along with cod-liver oil concentrates and all water-soluble vitamins, the concentrates to be used in large doses for a limited time, the high-vitamin-high-mineral diet to be kept up for life.

In the treatment for ulcers, Dr. Quigley expressly forbids all canned and packaged foods and use of white sugar and white flour products. He recommends milk, eggs, cheese, meat, raw fruit and vegetables, whole-wheat products, seafoods and vitamin and mineral supplements.

Now, remembering my intake of pineapple juice, see what Drs. J. D. Yeagley and D. Cayer reported in the *North Carolina Medical Journal* (November, 1948). Ulcer victims drinking orange juice had an increase in pain and burning sensations. The doctors suggested that, if citrus juice was given to ulcer patients, it should be in combination with other foods or at regular meal-time. Now you can see how wrong I was to drink cans and cans of pineapple juice, and on an empty stomach.

In 1950 the September issue of the *Journal of the American Dietetic Association* carried an article on the value of cabbage juice for ulcers. It was written by Dr. G. Cheney of the Department of Medicine of Stanford University. Dr. Cheney emphasized that the freshly made cabbage juice be taken in "small" quantities after other food had been taken. Again, note that juice was kept away from the empty stomach and the open ulcer crater.

Be Careful—In Choosing Your Vitamin C

I am convinced that vitamin C is needed in the healing process of an ulcer. But personal experience and medical literature indicate that citrus juices are not the way to get this needed vitamin C. Perhaps we have been oversold on juices. Furthermore, citrus fruit is not that rich in the vitamin. The average orange, grapefruit or lemon contains only 40 to 50 milligrams of vitamin C to every 100 grams of weight.

Vegetables like parsley, watercress, kale, collard

greens, turnip greens and broccoli have two to four times the amount of vitamin C. Parsley and watercress can be used frequently in salads. Kale, collard greens, turnip greens and broccoli should be steamed for a few minutes or pressure-cooked for a very brief time, barely enough to soften the fiber content. (Cooking these vegetables causes a loss of vitamins.) Or, if you prefer, especially with a denture problem, you may make a fresh vegetable drink from them in a blender. A few ounces of this green drink is permissible at the close of a meal. Adding some green cabbage to the mixture is optional.

I am not against an orange, two or three times a week, providing it is chewed, or half a grapefruit once a week. Occasional use of lemon juice on a salad is not detrimental. But to drink glasses of fruit juice, particularly citrus—definitely no.

Do have plenty of cantaloupe, papayas, mangoes, tangerines and tomatoes. These are almost as rich in vitamin C as oranges. Guavas have six times the amount. Rose-hips powder or tablets and acerola tablets have over twenty times as much vitamin C and won't sting or irritate the ulcer opening. Take the milder forms of vitamin C for your healing sources.

In addition, make sure you get enough of the highly protective proteins; these too are needed to repair tissue. Whole milk, soft-boiled or raw eggs, mild cheeses and lean meats are the more valuable proteins.

Cod-Liver Oil and Ulcers

In my own case, I found that the use of unrefined cod-liver oil mixed with a small amount of milk could keep me ahead of my ulcer. Unrefined cod-liver oil has a better natural quality of the essential fatty acids. This kind of oil has greater potential in the synthesis of new tissue. In spite of the effectiveness of fish oil, I find I can never again take carbonated drinks (not that I ever want to), juices, mustard, garlic, chives, scallion, black pepper, fresh pineapple and strong varieties of onion. Occasionally I do eat small amounts of the mild Spanish red onion and onion soups.

Accepted Treatment

Some eight and a half million Americans suffer from ulcers. Most of them have probably been told to stop worrying, that stress causes or irritates ulcers. My belief is that, at the most, worry plays a secondary role. Dietary mistakes are the primary cause. In this opinion, I am not alone.

An ulcer is always troublesome. At any point it can endanger the life of its victim. Hemorrhages and perforation of the gastric or duodenal wall are not too unusual.

If the ulcer progresses to the hemorrhage or per-foration stage, then the type of treatment demanded naturally varies with the severity of the disease. Close medical supervision is a must. Medical textbooks suggest the following diet:

1. **Milk, constantly at first. Must be used indefinitely.**
2. **Eggs are of major importance—raw, soft-boiled or poached.**
3. **Cooked cereals (milk types at first, then coarser kinds).**
4. **Fruits (pureed at first, no coarse seeds or skins, finally raw).**
5. **Vegetables (pureed at first, then steamed and finally raw).**
6. **Fresh meats (broiled ground beef, tender meats, chicken, fish. No dried, rolled, canned, spiced or processed meat).**

Protein and fat foods (correct types) are most desirable along with a high vitamin diet. Proteins combine readily with gastric secretions and reduce the need for free hydrochloric acid. Fats retard gastric secretions and delay passage of food from the stomach.

Alkali drugs (sodium bicarbonate) may be necessary to neutralize the gastric juices, temporarily.

Things to Avoid

1. **Highly seasoned foods.**
2. **Foods with coarse cellulose or tough fibers.**
3. **Foods that are chemically irritating to the ulcer. This means no caffeine foods like coffee and tea.**
4. **Gas-forming foods.**
5. **Extremely hot or extremely cold foods.**
6. **Sharply acid foods.**
7. **Alcoholic beverages.**
8. **Gravies.**
9. **Fruit juices.**
10. **White sugar and white flour.**
11. **Soft drinks of all types.**
12. **All devitalized foods.**

Ulcers take the joy out of eating. When you have to give up onion, you give up a remarkable ally. I was too late learning the value of this tremendous food, and then abused it.

Colitis

By definition, colitis means inflammation of the colon. There are two main types of colitis:

MUCOUS COLITIS: A condition manifested by tenderness of the abdomen, cramplike pains, alternating diarrhea and constipation. Emotional disturbance is blamed; I disagree.

ULCERATIVE COLITIS: A condition characterized by a severely inflamed colon, ulcerations and much pain. Diarrhea is always present, often 20 to 30 bloody stools a day. Obviously the body loses most of its proteins, fats, minerals, salts and water.

The constant need is to replace nutritional losses. A high-calorie, high-protein, high-vitamin, low-residue diet is recommended. The ulcerative-colitis sufferer presents one of the most difficult dietary problems in medicine.

It is believed the condition is basically one of infection and chemical irritations, with mental stresses generally thought to be present.

I believe, though, that ulcers, mucous colitis and ulcerative colitis are merely extensions of the same disease. Ulcers are probably early symptoms of colitis, and if the sufferer changes to a mild, bland diet, the latter generally can be avoided.

If dietary mistakes persist, even along with temporary control of the ulcer by using alkalis, the colon is going to suffer while the ulcer is being pacified. At this point colitis can be further aggravated by chemical irritants in food or drug intake, or by emotional upsets. But basically the same things that cause an ulcer, if continued, will have a major role in the cause of colitis.

In the bacterial forms of colitis, infection is enabled to get a start by a diet that causes malnutrition in the tissues. A diet of carbonated drinks, frozen juices, tea and devitalized foods affects the entire body. Spices and harsh vegetables add to the condition, and mental disturbances aggravate the situation even further.

How is bacterial infection of the colon triggered by poor diet? How can we say that ulcerated, infected intestines are caused by poor diet? Is there any scientific proof? Yes. Witness the challenging work of Dr. Paul Kouchakoff of the Institute of Clinical Chemistry of Lausanne, Switzerland.

In 1930 Dr. Kouchakoff described his work before the International Congress of Microbiology in Paris.

He discovered the startling fact that when the food eaten has been prepared at high temperatures or by complicated manufacturing processes, white blood cells appear in the intestinal tract. When an entire meal of raw, natural foods is eaten, no white blood cells appear. If, however, a person ate some cooked food or some devitalized foods, the effect could be neutralized by also taking some raw foods at the same meal.

Ordinarily, white blood cells are known to arise spontaneously at the site of an injury. Its function is to fight poisons and resist germs. Apparently chemical poisons exist in many refined foods. This leads to a creation of white blood cells in the intestinal flora, and soon these changes are reflected in the blood stream.

Dr. Kouchakoff believes that the presence or increase of white blood cells is an indication of some unhealthy process taking place because of this kind of food. White blood cells arrive in order to protect the body from harm. I think the appearance of microbes is then apparent. Here is your possible setting for bacterial infection.

This book and its beliefs are in agreement with Dr. Kouchakoff. I have said, over and over again, that devitalized foods lead to tissue malnutrition. The malnutrition gives way to degeneration which in turn yields to infection. My analysis has been stated simply, in laymen's terms, but Dr. Kouchakoff's work set forth the scientific meaning.

Much of this phenomenon occurs in seemingly unrelated diseases and disorders like rheumatoid arthritis, cancer, constipation and dandruff. Only the variation in strength of the different tissues determines where the degeneration, infection or bodily disturbance will take place.

The problem of ulcerative colitis is tragic. Often

it is a hopeless issue requiring surgical correction. Is it any wonder that textbooks give the impression that the disease is almost hopeless? Look at the diets they recommend. Their "Foundation Diets" (basic diet) for ulcerative colitis consist predominantly of refined foods. How can they expect results, in view of Dr. Kouchakoff's findings? His work is by-passed in nutritional research in this country.

I agree to the initial need for a bland diet. But those should be designed around natural, wholesome foods, not refined ones. Cod-liver oil is an excellent reparative food and at first should be used in very small amounts.

In my belief, ulcers and colitis can be controlled and prevented. Prevention is the better course; this I know through personal experience. Your kinds of dietary mistakes will differ from mine, so search out your incorrect eating habits and correct them.

If you persist with a bland diet of "refined foods," your chances of becoming constipated increase considerably. Let's take this opportunity to see how the problem of regulation can be sensibly controlled.

Chapter XVIII

Regularity Is Important . . . By Natural Means

When you start to follow a correct plan of diet—
as you select the proper foods and learn how to eat and
drink wisely—how soon will you notice an improvement
in your general health?

Some results of your better eating habits can be
expected quickly. Within a matter of days you should be
more alert . . . have more pep and energy . . . overcome
that "sluggish" and tired feeling which has slowed
down your entire body. For many people, one of the first
signs of improvement is their return to regularity, a vic-
tory over constipation.

Millions of Americans suffer from constipation. It
has been called "the disease of civilization." Primitive
people, as a group, were not constipated. Natives in re-
mote sections of the world today do not face this problem
of health. Why? Because they eat foods (meat, fish,
vegetables) that are not overrefined or overcooked,
many of them raw.

Yes, again in this case, civilization has made us
victims of overly processed and refined foodstuffs. I'm
certainly not going to recommend that, to defeat constipation, we all eat raw fish and discard all cooking tech-
niques. But we must develop a special set of eating habits

which will bring back the rhythm of evacuation within our intestinal tracts.

There are a number of "health foods"—organically grown products—which we can add to our daily diet to serve as a laxative. The safe way to remain regular is by natural means . . . and this chapter will tell you how.

Almost everyone experiences some degree of constipation at some period in his lifetime. That's why so many "cures" for this condition have been devised. You must learn to choose between a wide variety of commercially prepared laxatives. In fact, you must even avoid certain "home remedies" which cause harmful side effects.

The most popular fad for the relief of constipation is the practice of taking a mixture of lemon juice and water. This method will often work, temporarily. But, remember, fruit juices taken over a long period of time can create other health complications—problems far worse than being constipated. Throughout this book, I have emphasized that fruits should be eaten whole and that we should stay away from concentrated juices, because when you drink concentrated acid fruit juices you introduce the acids at too rapid a pace, without giving the digestive system sufficient time to neutralize them.

Prune juice is another favorite "laxative" used by people everywhere. Fortunately, it is the mildest of the fruit juices—and it will help for a time. Soon, however, the stimulative effect which prune juice has on your bowel muscle will wear off. For more lasting results, eat and chew organically grown unsulphured prunes.

Try these unsulphured prunes with your breakfast several times a week. As an alternate, for variety, eat unsulphured black mission figs. They have properties which make them an even better laxative. Eat these figs raw or pressure-cook them briefly. This suggestion can be important to anyone who has ulcers or colitis. Unsulphured black figs and prunes will do no harm to bodily oils.

Warm water, taken by itself, at least 30 minutes before breakfast is an effective aid to regularity. Drink two or three glasses, without the lemon juice.

Perhaps the best food product to combat constipation is raw wheat germ. Medical experiments have proven its value, and let me give you a typical example . . .

Dr. Robert McCarrison of Oxford, England, conducted a series of tests on monkeys. The bowel changes in the experimental monkeys were structurally and causally of the same nature as those found in chronically constipated arthritics. (When the monkeys were put on a bacteria-free diet, high in starches, their colons lost muscle tone and the membrane degenerated.)

This experiment was described in the *Journal of Laboratory and Clinical Medicine* by Dr. A. A. Fletcher of Toronto, Canada. Dr. Fletcher, in turn, set out to correct the problem of constipation in his human patients. He used raw wheat germ in his recommended diets. In addition, he tested the effect of wheat-germ extract and different forms of yeast.

To bring about improvement in the colon, the most successful product proved to be wheat germ.

My own experience indicates that raw wheat germ is far superior to the toasted varieties. I suggest that you use two tablespoons of raw wheat germ on your breakfast cereal, or sprinkle it on soup later in the day. Use it faithfully, but in these limited amounts.

There are some people with colitis who cannot tolerate wheat germ. For them, as a substitute, I suggest wheat germ flake cereal served with milk. The cereal is much milder, but it still serves as a laxative, and it is also a good source of vitamin B. To this cereal add some flake form brewers' yeast, a very important food supplement vital to regularity.

Bear in mind that there are dozens of brands of dry, boxed cereals on the market, most of which have been refined, processed and "fortified" with synthetic vitamins—but actually less than what was removed from the grain in the refining process. Such cereals do not completely meet the body's needs. Now better-quality dry cereals are obtainable in health-food stores and the more alert supermarkets. These include wheat germ flake, brown rice flake and bran and fig flake cereals.

A List of Foods to Help Regularity

If you are ready to agree that foods can relieve constipation by natural means, then let me give you an easy-reference guide. Here are several laxative-type foods, listed in the approximate order of their effectiveness . . .

1. Raw wheat germ
2. Brewers' yeast (flake-form)
3. Onions (mild, red, Spanish type, in moderation)
4. Scallions (in moderation)
5. Garlic (in moderation)
6. Figs (black, unsulphured)
7. Prunes (unsulphured, organically grown)
8. Dried fruits (apricots, in moderation)
9. Green celery
10. Cabbage (raw)
11. Cucumbers
12. Whole-wheat toast
13. Wheat germ flake cereal
14. Apples
15. Raisins
16. Raw carrots
17. Legumes
18. Lettuce (green)
19. Cauliflower (raw)
20. Spinach.

Many of the foods shown above are also included in the daily menus recommended in Chapter XX. They can help keep you free of constipation permanently. Commercially manufactured laxatives are, at best, only a temporary means of relief. Once you start to use such medicines, your body can become dependent on such artificial aid.

So, may I warn against the ten most common methods which are being used for "fast" results. . . .

Mineral oil. It's indigestible. It "surrounds" food particles when taken with a meal, and prevents your gaining value from elements in food (particularly vitamins).

Bran. Coarse grains may start clumping together in the intestinal tract, causing irritation of the digestive pathway.

Calomel. Causes added work for the liver.

Agar-agar. Envelops food particles with a film, so they are excreted before the proper food nutrients have been absorbed.

Cascara sagrada. Not always tolerated by your system, and it places an added strain on the liver.

Psyllium seeds. If they lodge in the intestinal walls, they become foreign irritants.

Cultured milk (buttermilk). Not nearly so effective as other methods, and gives strictly temporary results.

Senna. Creates more havoc for the congested liver. While removing waste, it also takes along with it some valuable digestive juices and food elements.

Milk of magnesia. A mild laxative, and not a lasting solution to the problem. However, this product at least does not do too much damage to bodily oils.

Colonic irrigations and enema. I believe that these methods should be confined to use in post-operative cases, in hospitals and just for the chronically ill.

All ten of the above remedies have one fault in common. They do not attack the basic cause of constipa-

tion. <u>They are merely emergency measures and con-</u>
<u>tribute nothing toward preventing a recurrence.</u>

For long-range protection against constipation we
must look to better diet and nature foods.

Brewers' yeast has been growing in popularity as
a laxative. This is one product which I do recommend.
It is a safer way, particularly for those who are troubled
with ulcers or colitis. Incidentally, if you suffer from
either of these conditions, let me inject a word of cau-
tion regarding raw onions and scallions. Don't overdo it
when eating these "sharp" vegetables, even though they
are on my approved list. You will find the red, Spanish
onion a much milder onion and the most easily tolerated
in the onion family.

Constipation Is an Illness in Itself

Too many people are inclined to minimize the fact
that they are occasionally constipated. They belittle the
danger and consider the situation as just a temporary
annoyance. Don't underestimate this phase of health.
Constipation is an actual "illness" . . . your body is fail-
ing to function properly.

There is even a set of "symptoms" which signal
this ailment. These signals may include fatigue, a coated
tongue, headaches, bad breath, skin blemishes and
nervousness.

More alarming is the fact that constipation is often
the prelude to a more serious disease. It may be a symp-

tom that you have something wrong somewhere in your body.

Therefore, I repeat, lack of regularity is a serious matter which you should not ignore. Do something about it! Correct your eating habits!

For your daily guidance, here is a list of seven simple rules:

1. For better digestion—and elimination later—chew each mouthful of food extremely well.

2. Avoid white sugar, sweets, refined foods, white bread. Through the years, they can cause a vitamin-B deficiency and a loss of bowel muscle tone.

3. For bulk in your diet, eat raw vegetables and fruits—organically grown, if possible.

4. Try to engage in some type of exercise every day. If not formal exercises, then straighten your back and pull in the muscles of your abdomen while you work. Try to improve your posture when you walk.

5. Set aside a regular time each day for evacuation.

6. If you miss one or two days, don't rush an artificially manufactured laxative into your system. Give nature's organically grown foods a chance to do their job.

7. Take long walks in the fresh air. Inhale deeply as you walk along. The added oxygen will help your metabolism.

By now, you can see that I favor a number of so-called health foods. Their value extends far beyond the problem of constipation. To show how they affect your health in general, I'll discuss the entire subject in the next chapter. . . .

Chapter XIX

There Is Good in Health Foods

Are health foods just a fad . . . a passing fancy from which the American public will soon turn away?

The answer is "No!" The preference for organically-grown foods—the widespread acceptance of vitamins, minerals and special food supplements—is here to stay. To augment your diet with health foods is highly beneficial. Millions of people are achieving results by learning to use natural foods as part of their daily meals, to compensate for the overrefinement of modern foods.

I have seen, from personal experience, the success which comes from eating fresh, organically grown fruits and vegetables. I visited a "health ranch" in Portersville, California, and also the ranch owned by Dr. H. E. Kirschner in Yucaipa, California. Dr. Kirschner is eighty years old, one of the last surviving doctors of his graduating class at Jefferson Medical College. He relies on organically grown food in his menus, and he insists that this is why he is outliving all his classmates.

Here was a doctor nearly twice my own age, yet he had more energy and "bounce" than I. We lived at the health ranch for three days, and he described to me the dietary habits which keep him well.

First, all foods grown there came from earth which

232

had never been contaminated by chemical fertilizers. Only natural fertilizers were used. As a result, the fruits and vegetables provided more enzymes and trace minerals—boron, copper, etc. Such foods also provide richer supplies of iron, calcium and phosphorus than foods produced under chemical fertilizer conditions.

Bread was baked, fresh, every morning. No additives were used in the bread, or in any other food. At the ranch, people also believed in taking vitamin-mineral supplements. But they made sure that these were natural (organic) vitamins and minerals which were extracted from living food sources.

Remember, your body does not manufacture the necessary vitamins and minerals. Therefore, you must gain your supply from outside sources . . . from foods or from special food supplements.

Some manufacturers of synthetic vitamins and minerals, instead of deriving the vitamins from living food sources, make capsules or potions by synthesizing inorganic chemicals (nonliving sources).

Synthetic vitamin A is often compounded with lemon grass oil, which in itself does not contain any vitamin A, to make substances called acetates or palmitates. These are fatty acids that resemble natural vitamin A except that they lack the necessary catalysts for complete assimilation. Much of the synthetic vitamin intake is lost in the urine, because it cannot be fully utilized in the body.

Another mistake is in the manufacture of synthetic

vitamin D—when it is created by ultra-violet ray irradiation. Compounded this way, the result is merely a product called ergosterol, which likewise lacks some essential complementary factors.

Synthetic vitamin C is generally made from processed corn sugar, and it lacks some of the important elements of natural vitamin C.

In all three of the above cases—which are typical —the synthetic vitamins reach the consumer with important factors missing. You have lost the helpful enzymes, unsaturated fatty acids and trace minerals.

So I repeat . . . if you are going to take artificially manufactured vitamins or other supplements, be certain they were derived from natural foods.

The United States Army also favors vitamins which come from foods. . . . Just read this quote from the official *United States Army Nutrition Manual*:

> Whenever possible, the nutrient required should be obtained from natural foods rather than synthetic preparations. This is particularly true of vitamins. Synthetic vitamin concentrates, tablets or pills may not contain all the known nutrients, either as such or in optimal proportion. Furthermore, they obviously may not contain lesser known or unknown nutrients which are, however, provided by natural foods.

Unfortunately, too many people are led astray by advertisements which promise a miracle vitamin pill. You may have heard TV commercials describing some pill "containing many vitamins," and how it is supposed

to satisfy all the daily requirements of your body. Nonsense.

It would be <u>impossible</u> to design a single unit capsule which would include all the necessary vitamins,
minerals, accessory factors, enzymes and life-giving
essentials. Your body requires different vitamins and
different minerals in different strengths—the bulk
quantities vary. The amount of one vitamin might be
measured in milligrams, while another is needed in
micrograms. Some elements you should receive in large
amounts, others in less concentrated form. No single
tablet can meet all these requirements.

While it is true that a limited number of enzymes
can be made synthetically, there are untold thousands
that science has not yet isolated, and <u>none</u> is incorporated in synthetic vitamin products.

Natural foods contain natural sources of these enzyme complexes.

The Best Sources of Natural Vitamins from Food Supplements

Instead of depending on some magic capsule, gain
better health the common-sense way. Here's a list of
recommended sources:

<u>Vitamin A and D</u>—from fish-liver oils.
<u>Vitamin B1 and B2 and many other B-complex
vitamins</u>—from brewers' yeast.

Vitamin C—from rose-hips extract and the acerola
   berry.
Vitamin E—from raw wheat germ.
Vitamin K—from soybean oil and leafy vegetables.

Regarding minerals, again you should seek out the
natural types. I suggest the following:

Iodine—from cod-liver oil and sea kelp.
Calcium—from sunflower seeds.
Phosphorus—from soya-lecithin.
Iron—from dessicated liver.
Manganese, Boron and Copper—from brewers'
   yeast.

Many of these foods do not have to be eaten "raw"
or whole. They, too, have been prepared into capsules,
tablets and bottled products. But the key fact is that the
vitamins and minerals have been extracted and derived
from natural sources. In general, I prefer the powdered,
granular or flake forms to the tablet or capsules because
they assimilate easier.

Health-food stores carry the largest assortment of
these items, but they are also available in some drug-
stores. It all comes down to reading the label . . . so you
can select your dietary supplements with their origin in
mind.

Before leaving this subject, let me state the best
advantage of all. When these natural supplements enter
the body, they are ready to go to work. Their physical

structure is right for the digestive system and they are immediately taken up by the tissues. Synthetic supplements, however—since they lack enzymes and complementary factors—require further synthesis from the body before they can be utilized.

How We "Preserve" Our Way Into Illness

One of the greatest dangers of modern living is the method we use to preserve our foods. I'm not attacking the old-fashioned practice of canning fruits and vegetables in glass jars. If you place certain garden products into jars, for use later in the winter, that's fine. But I am warning against the chemicals which some food manufacturers use as preservatives.

Highly processed foods—containing chemicals to color and preserve them—can have a ruinous effect on the enzymes in your body.

To understand this problem, let's examine the structure of a human body. Each of us is composed of billions of tiny units called cells. Each cell must "digest" food, excrete its wastes and repair itself. These reactions depend upon a chemical response which is triggered and controlled by a specific enzyme system.

Each cell contains from 50,000 to 100,000 of these enzyme systems—which are always ready to go to work in a millionth of a second.

Each enzyme system can be adversely affected by the merest trace of certain chemicals.

When the wrong preservatives are added to foods, they can upset the entire process of digestion.

Few people realize the extent of the threat from chemical preservatives. Do you realize that the average family in the United States could easily receive forty doses of these chemicals in one day? The best picture of this unhappy situation was prepared by a chemist working for the State of South Dakota. He compiled the following possible menu, to show you the hazards:

BREAKFAST

Canned cherries containing salicylic acid and coal-tar dye
Pancakes containing alum
Sausages containing borax and coal-tar dye
Syrup containing sodium sulphate
Baker's bread containing alum
Butter containing coal-tar dye

DINNER

Tomato soup containing benzoic acid and coal-tar dye
Corn scallops containing sulfurous acid and formalde-
   hyde
Pickles with copperas, sodium sulphate and salicylic acid
Corned beef and cabbage with saltpeter
Canned peas with salicylic acid
Vinegar with coal-tar dye
Catchup with benzoic acid and coal-tar dye
Lemon ice cream with methyl alcohol
Mince pie with boric acid

SUPPER

Canned beef with borax
Baked pork and beans with formaldehyde
Vinegar with coal-tar dye
Pickles with copperas, sodium sulphate and formalde-
   hyde
Catchup with coal-tar and benzoic acid
Bread and butter with alum and coal-tar dye

Lemon cake with alum
Cheese with coal-tar dye
Currant jelly with salicylic acid and coal-tar dye

The examples given above should be alarming enough to convince anyone of the health menace involved. Again, my purpose is not to conduct a "scare" campaign. I merely hope to awaken you—make you a little more cautious when you shop for groceries. Just read the labels on the food packages!

Federal laws require that the ingredients of food products be listed on the container. Read the small print!

Where the Health Food Industry Stands Today

As I travel across the United States on my lecture tours, I am more and more impressed by the number of health-food stores now appearing on the American scene. Public demand for natural foods is creating new businesses—new stores are being opened in cities everywhere.

I applaud this trend and predict that it will continue to grow. To supply the millions of health-food enthusiasts, new farms and ranches are now devoting more acres to organically grown products. Well-equipped laboratories have been built, to test and analyze the crops and to discover new benefits in foods.

With all this activity, how can critics call health foods "just a temporary fad"? The industry has become

a permanent asset to our country, a vital force in our
everyday life.

Merely because I favor health-food stores does not
mean that I endorse all their products. But these stores
do render a real service by making available certain
types of food supplements.

Which health foods do I particularly recommend?
Let me list a few of the best. . . .

BREWERS' YEAST is an excellent dietary aid. It
contains 16 of the 20 amino acids—forms of protein
which are necessary for your body to function properly.
Protein is needed for resistance to disease, for repair of
tissues and for longevity. Among the minerals found in
brewers' yeast are calcium, phosphorus, iron, potassium,
magnesium, silicon, sodium, zinc, manganese, copper,
iodine, lead, nickel and cobalt. What more can anyone
expect of any one food?

SOYA-LECITHIN can be extremely helpful. It provides your body with choline and inositol—two of the
B vitamins. This food, which is concentrated from soy-
beans, has the ability to emulsify fats. It helps reduce
blood cholesterol. Nutritionists believe that lecithin may
be a homogenizing agent—capable of breaking fat (and
probably cholesterol) into tiny particles which can pass
readily into the tissues.

(Some people will find the nutlike flavor of soya-
lecithin more palatable than brewers' yeast. However,
either product can be used on cereal or in soup without
losing its effectiveness. Personally, I add one to two

tablespoons of both flake-form brewers' yeast and soya-lecithin to my breakfast cereal.

RAW WHEAT GERM can be used also with brewers' yeast and soya-lecithin. Alternate these products, selecting raw wheat germ two or three times per week. It is a fine natural source of vitamins B and E. Your body needs vitamin E for reproduction and to help avoid sterility. A lack of vitamin E can also increase your susceptibility to heart disease, muscular disorders and paralysis.

DRIED FRUITS in your diet should include black mission figs and black prunes—sold in health food stores in bags marked "unsulphured." (Too often, dried fruits have been sprayed with sulphur or other preservatives.) Another good choice would be dried apricots and organically grown raisins—such as the Monuka variety. Use these fruits on top of your breakfast cereal, and serve it with room-temperature milk. These same dried fruits can also be eaten as snacks between meals.

In our own home we use brown rice flake cereal, wheat germ flake cereal, bran and fig flake cereal and wheat flake cereal. These varieties are generally sold in health food stores. One of them may appeal to you.

At breakfast, to the dry cereal we occasionally add unsulphured fruits. After half of the cereal-fruit combination is eaten, we add the brewers' yeast and soya-lecithin or raw wheat germ. Cereal is used about three times a week.

In colder weather we enjoy a warm cereal—like

wheat and soya cereal. Then, for a change, we have millet seed cereal or oatmeal.

Many of the foods I have just described will be found in the menus in Chapter XX. Please remember that these products are recommended as dietary supplements . . . they are not intended to replace all the more commonly known foods. I am not suggesting that you try to exist entirely on health foods. There is no need to take radical measures, just give your meals some added support through the use of these special items in moderate amounts two or three times a week.

No matter how many "health foods" you consume, you must continue your vigilance in other areas of nutrition. Even organically grown foods will suffer from overcooking and overbaking. If you allow fresh vegetables to wilt—or fruits to turn color—before eating them, then you have already lost some of their enzymatic value.

Yes, the people who eat health foods often make the same mistakes. They forget about proper methods of food preparation—and neglect other rules at mealtime. So, to remind everyone of the correct course, the next chapter will feature complete menus.

Chapter XX

Recommended Menus: Your Day-by-Day Guide

INCLUDING A NUMBER OF NATURAL FOOD
SUPPLEMENTS FOR VITAMINS AND MINERALS

For the past nineteen chapters we have explored a wide range of foods and dietary supplements. There have been specific recommendations for specific maladies. However, this chapter lists menus recommended for all. *Everyone who seeks vital health and good body tone will do well to follow these menus.* Now, a good question arises. "What happens when we try to combine all these different food elements into the same meal?"

Perhaps you suspect by now that the result would be a drab, tasteless diet. On the contrary, I have good news. It is perfectly possible to observe all the rules of good nutrition and still enjoy your meals. The foods recommended in this book do have taste appeal and variety.

Good eating is one of the great joys of life. And of course, so is good health. You can have both simply by maintaining the proper balance of liquids and solids in your diet. All it takes is a little preplanning.

As an example—a typical guide for you to follow

—the next few pages contain actual menus. Here is an outline, day by day, for an entire week. In these menus you will find familiar foods, new foods and some natural supplements which can add value to your daily diet. After you have tried this "bill of fare" for a few days, use the same pattern to design your own meals. Develop your own long-range dietary plan.

Remember one important consideration. Check your weight before selecting a set of menus. If you are overweight or underweight, modify your diet accordingly. This list of meals shows you how. Turn the page and . . . Bon Appétit!

SEVEN DAYS OF RECOMMENDED MENUS

FOR PEOPLE OF NORMAL WEIGHT

MONDAY

BREAKFAST

Egg (boiled) 1 (3-minute)
Cottage cheese ... ½ cup
Rye or corn bread. 1 slice
Butter .... 1 pat
Prunes (raw) 3-4
Milk .... 8 oz.
Vitamin-mineral tablet
  (take with milk)

LUNCH

Fruit salad plate: sliced banana, apple,
  raisins and peaches
Melba toast
Milk .... 8 oz.

DINNER

Tomato soup ..... 1 cup
Steak (broiled) .. large serving
Baked potato..... medium
Butter .... 1 pat
Choice of fruit
Milk .... 8 oz.

9 P.M.—11 P.M.
Celery sticks with cream cheese
  (optional)

TUESDAY

BREAKFAST

Stewed prunes and apricots
Wheat flake cereal 1 bowl
Brewers' yeast
  (flake-form) ... 2 tbsp.
Kelp granules .... ½ tsp.
Soya-lecithin
  granules .... 1 tbsp.
Rose-hips powder. ½ tsp.
  (Mix four ingredients above into
  last portion of cereal)
Milk .... 8 oz.

LUNCH

Shrimp salad .... 4-6 shrimp
Green lettuce
  leaves 3-4
Carrot sticks
Choice of fruit
Milk .... 8 oz.

DINNER

Vegetable soup... 1 cup
Meat loaf with hard-boiled egg
Lima beans ...... ½ cup
Lettuce and tomato salad
Berries (in season) or choice of fruit
Milk .... 8 oz.

9 P.M.—11P.M.
Choice of fresh fruit
  (optional)

WEDNESDAY

BREAKFAST

Oatmeal .... 1 cup
Raw wheat germ.. 1 tbsp.
 (Mix into oatmeal when served)
Figs (black,
  unsulphured) .. 2-3
Milk .... 8 oz.

LUNCH

Chicken liver omelet
Green beans ..... ½ cup
Asparagus .... ½ cup
Apple .... 1 large
Milk .... 8 oz.

DINNER

Shrimp cocktail... 3-4 shrimp
Tossed green salad
Liver (broiled) .. 6 oz.
Fresh spinach .... ½ cup
Steamed onions .. ¼ cup
Melon in season
Milk .... 8 oz.

10 P.M.—11 P.M.
COD-LIVER OIL MIXTURE
 (Taken and mixed as described in
 Chapter XIII)

THURSDAY

BREAKFAST

Sliced orange 1
Poached eggs on whole-wheat toast
Cottage cheese ... ½ cup
Milk .... 8 oz.
Vitamin-mineral tablet
 (take with milk)

LUNCH

Fresh fruit plate (sliced banana, ½
  sliced pear, small bunch of grapes,
  1 sliced apple, ¼ cup raisins)
Melba toast or zwieback
Milk .... 8 oz.

DINNER

Lentil soup ...... 1 cup
Roast beef (lean). 6-8 oz.
Succotash .... ½ cup
Lettuce and tomato salad
Cantaloupe or choice of fruit
Milk .... 8 oz.

9 P.M.—11 P.M.
Carrot sticks
 (optional)

FRIDAY

BREAKFAST

Choice of dry cereal (bran and fig flake, wheat flake or brown rice flake)

Brewers' yeast
(flake-form) ... 2 tbsp.

Soya-lecithin
granules .... 1 tbsp.

Rose-hips powder. ½ tsp.

Kelp granules .... ½ tsp.
(Mix four ingredients above into last half-portion of cereal)

Milk .... 8 oz.

LUNCH

Baked salmon .... 4-6 oz.

Lima beans ...... ½ cup

Beets .... ½ cup

Nectarine or apple

Milk .... 6 oz.

DINNER

Fish chowder .... 1 cup

Choice of meat or fish

Tossed salad

Fresh fruit cocktail

Milk .... 8 oz.

10 P.M.—11 P.M.

COD-LIVER OIL MIXTURE

SATURDAY

BREAKFAST

Ham and eggs

Rye bread (toast) 2 slices

Butter .... 1 pat

Prunes or figs.... 3-4

Milk .... 8 oz.

Vitamin-mineral tablet
(take with milk)

LUNCH

Cold meat sandwich

Baked beans ..... ½ cup

Sliced tomato .... 2-3 slices

Milk .... 6-8 oz.

DINNER

Bean and barley
soup .... 1 cup

Lamb chops or
veal cutlet ..... 6-8 oz.

Boiled potato (in jacket)

Grated carrot and celery salad

Melon in season.. ½

Milk .... 8 oz.

9 P.M.—11 P.M.

Apple
(optional)

SUNDAY

BREAKFAST
Canadian bacon or lean ham
Eggs (poached) .. 2
Corn or rye bread. 1 slice
Butter .... 1 pat
Banana
Milk .... 8 oz.

SUPPER
Grilled cheese sandwich
Fresh fruit cup
Milk .... 8 oz.

DINNER
Minestrone soup.. 1 cup
Choice of roast chicken or turkey
Cranberry sauce
Celery sticks and black olives
String beans ..... ½ cup
Fruit or melon in season
Milk .... 8 oz.

9 P.M.—11P.M.

Banana
   (optional)

SEVEN DAYS OF RECOMMENDED MENUS

FOR PEOPLE WHO ARE UNDERWEIGHT

MONDAY

BREAKFAST
Oatmeal .... 1 cup
Raw wheat germ.. 1 tbsp.
   (Mix with oatmeal when served)
Egg (soft-boiled). 1
Pumpernickel or
   rye bread ...... 1 slice
Butter .... 1 pat
Milk .... 10 oz.
Vitamin-mineral tablet
   (take with milk)

LUNCH
Bean and barley
   soup .... 1 cup
French toast ..... 2 slices
Cottage cheese ... 1 cup
Fresh fruit cup
Milk .... 10 oz.

DINNER
Steak (broiled)... large serving
Baked potato..... 1 large
Salad (lettuce, tomato, radishes, car-
   rots, celery and cucumber)
Banana 1
Milk .... 10 oz.

7:00 P.M.—7:30 P.M.
Milk .... 10 oz.
Pepita seeds 40-50

10 P.M.—11 P.M.
COD-LIVER OIL MIXTURE

TUESDAY

BREAKFAST

Pumpernickel toast 2 slices
Egg (boiled) .... (3-minute)
Choice of fresh fruit cup or melon
Brown rice flake cereal
Brewers' yeast
    (flake-form) ... 2 tbsp.
Soya-lecithin
    granules .... 1 tbsp.
Kelp granules .... ½ tsp.
Rose-hips powder. ½ tsp.
    (Mix four ingredients above into
    last half-portion of cereal)
Milk .... 10 oz.

LUNCH

Beef stew .... 1 bowl
Tossed green salad
Banana or apple.. large
Milk .... 10 oz.

DINNER

Hamburger patties
    (broiled) ..... 2 large
Potato, mashed
Tomato 1
Corn .... 1 cup
Melon or fruit in season
Milk .... 10 oz.

7:00 P.M.—7:30 P.M.

Milk .... 10 oz.
Sunflower seeds... 40-50
Vitamin-mineral
    emulsion tonic.. 1 tbsp.

WEDNESDAY

BREAKFAST

Wheat and soya
    cereal .... 1 cup
Raw wheat germ.. 2 tbsp.
Raisin bread
    (toast) .... 2 slices
Butter .... 1 pat
Stewed apricots, prunes and figs
Milk .... 10 oz.
Vitamin-mineral tablet
    (take with milk)

LUNCH

Green pea soup... 1 bowl
Minute steak and beans
Choice of fruit
Milk .... 10 oz.

DINNER

Veal cutlet
    (baked) ...... 8 oz.
Baked potato..... large
Butter .... 1 pat
Celery and cheese sticks
Apple and raisin salad
Milk .... 10 oz.

7:00 P.M.—7:30 P.M.

Milk .... 10 oz.
Pepita seeds 40-50

10 P.M.—11 P.M.

COD-LIVER OIL MIXTURE

THURSDAY

BREAKFAST

Egg (poached) .. 1
Whole-grain bread 1 slice
Butter .... 1 pat
Choice of good-grade dry cereal
Brewers' yeast
 (flake-form) ... 2 tbsp.
Kelp granules .... ½ tsp.
Soya-lecithin
 granules .... 1 tbsp.
Rose-hips powder. ½ tsp.
 (Mix four ingredients above into
 last half-portion of cereal)
Stewed prunes ... 3-4
Milk .... 10 oz.

LUNCH

Cheese and nut sandwich
Fresh fruit cup
Milk .... 10 oz.

DINNER

Tomato and brown rice soup
Baked meat loaf
 and hard-boiled
 egg .... 1 slice
Asparagus .... ½ cup
Grated carrot and raisin salad
Banana
Milk .... 10 oz.

7:00 P.M.—7:30 P.M.

Milk .... 10 oz.
Sunflower seeds .. 40-50
Vitamin-mineral
 emulsion tonic.. 1 tbsp.

FRIDAY

BREAKFAST

Choice of toast,
 buttered ...... 1-2 slices
Wheat germ flake cereal
Raw wheat germ.. 2 tbsp.
Cottage cheese and
 banana .... 1 cup
Milk .... 10 oz.
Vitamin-mineral tablet
 (take with milk)

LUNCH

Scallops, baked on
 skewer .... 6-8 scallops
Sweet potato ..... medium
String beans ..... ½ cup
Milk .... 10 oz.

DINNER

Shrimp cocktail .. 4-6 shrimp
Lobster (broiled)
Corn .... 1 cup
Carrots and raisin salad
Fruit cup (apples, peaches, pears and
 cherries)
Milk .... 10 oz.

7:00 P.M.—7:30 P.M.

Milk .... 10 oz.
Dried fruit of your choice

10 P.M.—11 P.M.

COD-LIVER OIL MIXTURE

SATURDAY

BREAKFAST

Buckwheat
    pancakes 3
Butter .... 2 pats
Maple syrup ..... 2 tbsp.
Cottage cheese ... 1 cup
Milk .... 10 oz.

LUNCH

Seafood casserole
Tomato and cucumber salad
Hard roll
Apple .... 1 large
Milk .... 10 oz.

DINNER

Oysters or clams
Liver (broiled)
    and onions ..... large portion
Baked potato and butter
Steamed carrots... 1 cup
Pear or apple..... 1 large
Milk .... 10 oz.

7:00 P.M.—7:30 P.M.

Milk .... 10 oz.
Pepita seeds 40-50
Vitamin-mineral
    emulsion tonic... 1 tbsp.

SUNDAY

BREAKFAST

Bacon and eggs
Corn bread ...... 2 slices
Choice of melon or prunes
Cottage cheese ... 1 cup
Milk .... 10 oz.
Vitamin-mineral tablet
    (take with milk)

SUPPER

Bowl of chicken broth
Meat sandwich
Tossed green salad
Milk .... 10 oz.

DINNER

Chicken or steak (broiled)
Mashed potato
Fresh spinach .... 1 cup
Carrot curls
Celery and cheese sticks
Milk .... 10 oz.

7:00 P.M.—7:30 P.M.

Milk .... 10 oz.
Pepita seeds 40-50
Vitamin-mineral
    emulsion tonic.. 1 tbsp.

SEVEN DAYS OF RECOMMENDED MENUS

FOR PEOPLE WHO ARE OVERWEIGHT

MONDAY

BREAKFAST

Oatmeal .... ½ cup
Raw wheat germ.. 2 tbsp.
Milk .... 6 oz.
Vitamin-mineral tablet
  (take with milk)

LUNCH

Cheese sandwich
Carrot curls
Pear .... medium
Milk .... 6 oz.

DINNER

Consommé ...... 1 cup
Roast beef (lean). 4 oz.
Tomato and lettuce salad
Coleslaw
Apple .... 1 medium
Milk .... 6 oz.

9 P.M.—11 P.M.

One celery stick
  (optional)

TUESDAY

BREAKFAST

Poached eggs on whole-wheat toast
Choice of prunes or apricots
Milk .... 6 oz.

LUNCH

Clear soup .... 1 cup
Hamburger
  (broiled) ...... medium
Coleslaw .... 1 cup
Milk .... 6 oz.

DINNER

Steamed carrots .. 1 cup
Fresh spinach .... 1 cup
Celery sticks
Lima beans ...... ½ cup
Choice of fruit in season
Milk .... 6 oz.

9 P.M.—11 P.M.

Apple
  (optional)

WEDNESDAY

BREAKFAST

Pumpernickel or
   rye bread ...... 1 slice
Egg (soft-boiled). 1
Milk .... 6 oz.
Vitamin-mineral tablet
   (take with milk)

LUNCH

Melon or fresh fruit cup
Cottage cheese ... 1 cup
Melba toast
Milk .... 6 oz.

DINNER

Salmon salad
Carrot and raisin salad on lettuce
Succotash
Pear or banana
Milk .... 6 oz.

9 P.M.—11 P.M.

Three carrot sticks
   (optional)

THURSDAY

BREAKFAST

Prunes (raw or
   stewed) 3 4
Egg (soft-boiled) . 1 (3-minute)
Melba toast
Milk .... 6 oz.

LUNCH

Sliced hard-boiled eggs on lettuce
Tomato, celery, carrot salad
Cottage cheese ... ½ cup
Milk .... 6 oz.

DINNER

Bouillon .... 1 cup
Ry-krisp 2
Lettuce and tomato salad
Steak (broiled) .. 6 oz.
Green peas ...... ½ cup
Milk .... 6 oz.

9 P.M.—11 P.M.

Apple
   (optional)

FRIDAY

BREAKFAST
Wheat germ flake cereal
Brewers' yeast
(flake-form) ... 2 tbsp.
Soya-lecithin
granules .... 1 tbsp.
Kelp granules .... ½ tsp.
Rose-hips powder. ½ tsp.
(Mix four ingredients above into
last half-portion of cereal)
Milk .... ½ glass

DINNER
Salmon (broiled). 4 oz.
Baked potato..... ½
Butter .... ½ pat
Green celery ..... 2 stalks
Apple .... medium
Milk .... 6 oz.

LUNCH
Hamburger (broiled) on roll
Cottage cheese and green lettuce leaves
Milk .... 6 oz.

10 P.M.—11 P.M.
COD-LIVER OIL MIXTURE
(Taken and mixed as described in
Chapter XIII)

SATURDAY

BREAKFAST
Fresh orange slices
Choice of cereal.. ½ cup
Choice of raw
wheat germ or
brewers' yeast
(flake-form) ... 2 tbsp.
Milk .... 6 oz.
Vitamin-mineral tablet
(take with milk)

DINNER
Roast beef (lean and medium-rare)
Tossed green salad
Corn .... ½ cup
Milk .... 6 oz.

LUNCH
Vegetable salad (tomato, lettuce, car-
rots, green peppers, cucumber)
Choice of dressing, small amount
Melba toast
Milk .... 6 oz.

9 P.M.—11 P.M.
1 or 2 bread dates
(optional)

SUNDAY

BREAKFAST	DINNER
Whole-wheat toast (buttered)	Vegetable soup ... 1 cup
Ham and egg	Steak (broiled)... 8 oz.
Prunes 2-3	Carrot sticks 2-3
Milk .... 6 oz.	Broccoli .... ½ cup
Vitamin-mineral tablet	Milk .... 6 oz.
(take with milk)	

SUPPER

Fruit salad (peaches, apples, prunes
and cottage cheese)
Milk .... 6 oz.

9 P.M.—11 P.M.

Apple or banana
(optional)

The menus in this chapter have started you on a new adventure in good eating. They have pointed the way to better health.

On your own, you can make changes, alternate the foods to different days of the week, etc. For variety of food choice, see Chapter XIII. Just maintain the same general plan, the pattern. As your reward, you will soon feel livelier, more alert and more confident. Your body will be building a strong resistance to many types of disease.

In the matter of salad dressings, use your favorite kind, but in very small amounts (about 1 teaspoonful per individual serving). This should apply to whatever oil you use on your salad. It is our opinion that the good or harm that the salad oil will contribute is controlled by the choice of liquid with the meal. Free use of vinegar is not approved.

I know that these menus will produce results. They were devised in a manner similar to the menus used against arthritis. Thousands of arthritics have used a dietary approach to their problem. I forecast that you will have equal success when you put these new menus to work to combat or prevent other illnesses. I predict that these meals and nutritional rules will stand the test of time . . . will face any clinical evaluation and prove their worth!

Chapter XXI

Clinical Proof Supports This Dietary Plan

In the world of science and research, no discovery really counts until it has been clinically tested. Until a hospital, laboratory or group of doctors has officially studied a new theory, it will not be accepted by organized medicine.

In order to meet the properly very high standards set by the American Medical Association, the chief arbiter of matters relating to our nation's health, any new treatment or medical theory must be thoroughly tested in clinics or hospitals. Findings must be corroborated by clinical investigators independent of the originator of the treatment or theory.

But I must point out that too often it is very difficult to arrange testing by a recognized clinic. For five consecutive years, I urged medical scientists to make a clinical evaluation of my dietary program for arthritics. Time and again, members of the profession declined—refused even to consider that diet might alleviate arthritis.

Finally, in the summer of 1957, I was able to arrange a formal test of my dietary regimen. The project was conducted by the Brusch Medical Center, Cambridge, Massachusetts. The clinical evaluation was under

257

the supervision of Dr. Charles A. Brusch and Dr. Edwin T. Johnson. They and the staff at the Medical Center worked for many months to determine the importance of diet as a weapon against this chronic disease.

Now we are ready to announce the results.

So that you can appreciate the significance of this clinical evaluation, I would like to describe it in detail. When you see the progress achieved by actual patients, use your own judgment about the value of good nutrition.

As you read the history of what happened at the clinic, certain facts will become clear immediately. Notice the close parallels—the interesting comparisons —with everything we have been discussing in this book. The same type of dietary plan was followed. The same "liquids versus solids" rules were applied. The same restrictions were placed against the use of soft drinks, white sugar and other foods I have described in this book as unsatisfactory and detrimental.

This clinical study began in July, 1957, and continued until January, 1958. Included in the tests were ninety-eight unselected cases of arthritis coming through the Medical Center for treatment. All were placed on my dietary regimen.

Osteo, rheumatoid and mixed types of arthritis were treated—including cases in the early, moderate and severe stages.

Basically, the therapeutic criteria of the American Rheumatism Association were followed.

Of the patients participating in our tests, some 40 per cent of them had been X-rayed. There was a preponderance of Class 2 (moderately severe) cases.

In all cases, blood and urine samples were drawn at the start and periodically for comparative study.

Sedimentation rates, cholesterol levels, complete blood counts and urinalysis were studied on all patients. Where necessary, blood sugar levels were determined.

Some 25 per cent of the study group had, at some time in the past, been treated with steroid hormones, gold salts, paraffin-wax baths and aspirin—without success.

During the study no subjects used steroid hormones, gold salts or paraffin-wax baths.

About 58 per cent of the group had been receiving either liver-iron supplements or physiotherapy without significant improvement prior to the study. These patients continued taking vitamins, minerals, aspirin and heat treatments while following the dietary regimen we prescribed.

AT THE START OF THE CLINICAL EVALUATION . . .

1. 68 per cent of the patients exhibited some degree of dry skin, scalp and hair. Simultaneously, brittle fingernails were a frequent occurrence—particularly among women.
2. 43 per cent were negative for earwax.
3. 58 per cent had moderate to pronounced swelling beneath the eyes.
4. 67 per cent had dentures.
5. 23 per cent had poor complexion.
6. 19 per cent were constipated regularly or iregularly.
7. 15 per cent had impaired hearing.

We pursued a course to substantiate our belief that most arthritic problems have their basis to a large degree in diet and eating habits.

It was felt that both degenerative and proliferative arthritis could be resolved through a modified dietary regimen.

We classified together rheumatoid, osteo and gouty arthritis in a single clinical study. One reason we took this course is that all these forms of arthritis have a common denominator called "blood sludge."

Among all the patients the only new element introduced was our dietary regimen. They followed our plan of diet—and their reactions were observed—over a period of approximately six months.

THE SYSTEM OF DIET CONTROL

1. Water was consumed upon arising, preferably at warm temperatures and about 60 minutes before breakfast. (Additional water was allowed 30 minutes before the evening meal.)
2. Room-temperature milk (whole or homogenized), or warm soup (not creamed) were the only liquids permitted with meals. These two liquids were permitted at any meal. Acceptable solids were permitted at any time of the day, providing they were not accompanied by the wrong liquids.
3. Cod-liver oil, mixed with either two tablespoons of fresh, strained orange juice or two tablespoons of milk, was taken on a fasting stomach—four or preferably five or more hours after the evening meal or before retiring; or one or more hours before breakfast, and at least 30 minutes after water intake. The oil was taken daily. (Where there were dietary complications or accompanying conditions—like diabetes or heart disease—it was taken only two times a week to facilitate assimilation. It has been found that peo-

ple with these conditions take to the regimen easier this way.)

The cod-liver oil and milk mixture—especially for advanced sensitive arthritics—is preferable to the orange juice mixture.

4. There was complete elimination of soft drinks, candy, cake, pie, ice cream or any food made up of white sugar.
5. Those who felt that the sacrifice of coffee was too great were allowed black coffee following the water intake in the morning upon arising, providing it was taken at least 15 minutes before breakfast.
6. The diets recommended for the subjects ranged from 1,800 to 2,400 calories.

Throughout this clinical evaluation, a special interrogation chart was used. Its purpose was to elicit complete information about the patient. The complete background of all liquid intake, its temperature and the time of intake, was recorded.

The same questionnaire routine was applied to every detail in the solid portion of the meal. Complete objective data (on the condition of each patient's skin, scalp, hair, ears and nails) were detailed into the charts from the physical examination.

The Doctors Report

Here are the findings, the final report made at the end of the clinical evaluation, as published in the July, 1959, issue of the *Journal of the National Medical Association*. These facts were established, and I now quote Dr. Brusch and Dr. Johnson:

Ninety-two per cent of the patients responded to the dietary regimen within periods of 2 to 20 weeks. . . .

Subjectively, this consisted of <u>marked reduction of pain and general improvement in well-being</u> in the majority of patients.

Objectively, there was diminished tissue swelling, improved range of motion and mobility, less fatigue, better complexion, frontal [forehead] signs of luster, skin and scalp improvement, re-established levels of cerumen [earwax], stronger nails, and much more alertness.

[You can imagine my thrilled reaction when I read these statements for the first time. It was the most gratifying experience of my life—to have clinical proof of what I had already learned, that my dietary research was correct and could help millions of arthritics. Now let's return to Drs. Brusch and Johnson and their Summary Report. . . .]

Favorable changes in blood chemistry consistently occurred in conjunction with definite clinical improvement in over 90 per cent of the cases.

The data obtained and observations made in this study strongly suggest that further research along these lines is indicated and that further exploration of the relationship between diet and adrenal function may prove most fruitful.

The two typical case histories reproduced below are actual records from the Medical Center. They represent just two of the many patients who gained better health.

ACTUAL CASE HISTORIES
(from the Clinical Evaluation of our Dietary Regimen)

CASE 22: Male. July 22, 1957.
<u>Condition before dietary treatment:</u>

Three years ago both shoulders and elbows became painful. Out of work for 18 months. Asymptomatic until six weeks ago when there was onset of pain in low back, right hip and right knee. In bed for two weeks. Has morning stiffness occasionally over entire body. Is subject to weather changes. Feet frequently cold in summer. Tongue slightly coated. Poor oral hygiene. Weight 189½.

Nails brittle, neck was pronounced wrinkling, skin dry, encrustations of the eyes, symmetrical pouches beneath the eyes, scalp itchy and dry. Ears negative for earwax.

Blood chemistry: Sedimentation rate 5. Cholesterol 280. Blood sugar 115.

X-ray findings: compression of the superior plate of L 2 with narrowing of the disc space L 1-2. Minimal degenerative arthritic changes in lumbar spine. Marked calcification of the abdominal aorta is noted.

Diagnosis: Osteoarthritis.

Diet prescribed:

Lemon juice with brown sugar and skimmed milk eliminated. Water-drinking habits corrected. Whole milk suggested at all meals. Cod-liver oil mixed with orange juice four times a week, later to be changed to cod-liver oil with milk.

Follow-up examinations:

Patient subsequently seen on 10 different occasions during a five-month period. Patient discharged on December 28, 1957.

Results:

Reduction in sedimentation rate from 5 to 1. Cholesterol decreased 10 mg. per 100 cc.'s of blood.

Skin, scalp, hair and nails all improved. Ears, which were negative for earwax, now have a moderate amount.

Patient no longer complains of painful joints.

CASE 120: Female. September 6, 1957.

Condition before dietary treatment:

Pain in cervical vertebrae for past 4 to 5 years. No changes in symptoms except pain radiating to thoracic region. Swelling of right knee at onset of menopause (age 52).

Externally, skin is dry. Moderate wrinkling of the neck. Ears dry and inflamed. Nails brittle. Patient is edentulous [toothless].

Blood chemistry: Sedimentation rate 17. Cholesterol 388. Blood sugar 102.

X-ray findings: C-spine. Marked degenerative arthritis with compression of the bodies of C 5 and C 6 at the intervertebral foramina at these levels bilaterally. The body of C 3 lies 3 mm. anterior D—C 4. A spondylolisthesis, probably secondary D degenerative changes. Moderately advanced degenerative arthritic changes are noted in the bones of the right knee.

Diagnosis: Marked osteoarthritis.

Diet prescribed:

Chronic imbiber of tea and soft drinks. Diet was corrected. Cod-liver oil regimen was instituted three times a week.

Follow-up examinations:

Subsequently seen on six different occasions during a 14-week period. Patient discharged on December 30, 1957.

Results:

Marked reduction in sedimentation rate to 9. Cholesterol decreased 50 mg. per 100 cc. of blood. Blood sugar level lower at 100 mg. per 100 cc. of blood.

Skin texture improved, scalp has more natural oils.

Asymptomatic with no complaints.

In no way did the prescribed dietary regimen interfere with previously instituted therapies. Rather, our findings indicate that the effectiveness of chemotherapy and physiotherapy is enhanced by the addition of the dietary program prescribed by the authors.

The authors feel their objective and subjective findings suggest that adherence to their prescribed regimen on a long-term basis will result in sustained clinical improvement.

CHARLES A. BRUSCH, M.D.
EDWARD T. JOHNSON, M.D.

Additional Comments and Observations

The final report prepared by the Medical Center was 19 pages long. Here, in this book, I have condensed the material and have covered only the highlights. But I have reproduced enough of the report so that you can see the resounding success of this clinical test.

I would like to summarize a few other results which were most impressive to me. At the conclusion of the six-month clinical study, the patients also showed these improvements:

1. Sedimentation rates dropped consistently.
2. Cholesterol levels dropped, or could be controlled, even with the introduction of milk, eggs, butter and cod-liver oil.
3. High white blood cell counts gave way to normal white blood cell counts.
4. Hemoglobin levels frequently went up. Increases of 0.4 to 1.6 grams per 100 cc. of blood above prestudy levels were noted when the hemoglobin level had originally been below normal.
5. Blood sugar levels turned to the lower side of normal.
6. Blood pressure levels were found to be lower, after 10 to 15 weeks.
7. Body weight remained almost static.

8. Acid urines remained acid, but alkaline urines became acid.

9. A phenomenon known as urinary mucous threads generally cleared. (I believe the presence of mucous threads in urine sediment reflects active mental stress.)

As an average, within three months dry skin, scalp and hair were corrected by the diet and returned to more normal conditions. This also held true regarding the replacement of earwax.

Improvements in complexion were impressive.

Constipation was gradually overcome.

The majority of the patients evidenced increased warmth in their extremities, less swelling and more energy, after four to five months on the regimen.

Perhaps the information in this chapter has opened your eyes, too. At last—through this clinical evaluation —we have substantial proof. No one can deny this evidence, this record of performance among actual patients. And we can expand the findings of this plan of nutrition to the entire field of general health. Furthermore, you can apply the principles to your own daily life.

Chapter XXII

A Challenge for the Future

And now I want to remind you of the points I made at the very beginning of this book. You are the only one who can hold the key to your good health, and the name of that key is Common Sense.

The beginning of wisdom about your health is to know the state of your health. Of course the best method is to have a complete physical examination by your own physician. A closely observed "clinical evaluation" is an excellent idea for any person even if he does not feel ill.

But health and well-being are ever-changing. You have to keep on guard. You have to keep checking on your health. I believe that it is possible to check your own body . . . you can at least learn to recognize certain symptoms. You can tell, in advance, the preliminary signs of many illnesses. This knowledge—this ability to recognize symptoms—can be your best safeguard for the future. As soon as you see symptoms or feel the onslaught of an ailment, go to your doctor and accurately describe your condition. Discuss it, and he can then give you the necessary examination.

Your future course—your personal campaign for better health—is now a challenge which you must face alone. The opportunity is yours. This book has given you a plan of action—a detailed guide which you must now choose to follow or ignore.

The dietary regimen proposed in these pages can start you on a new way of life. A better, healthier, happier way.

But to work effectively, the suggestions and recommendations we have made must become part of your daily schedule. If you plan to observe these rules of diet on just a part-time basis, forget it. You will gain little value from an "occasional" use of these menus. Halfway measures will not solve an important issue like personal health.

Yes, you now face a real challenge. Do you have the strength and determination to practice what you have learned? Will you revise your eating habits, test these new theories, give them a fair trial? I believe that you will.

All anyone can ask is that you <u>try</u> this plan of proper nutrition and stay with it long enough to notice the results. When you begin to feel better—when you <u>feel</u> the improvement in your own body—there will be no question about your continuing on this correct road to a longer life.

Though you will be practicing good nutrition by yourself, millions of others may soon join you in the same approach. More and more doctors are recommending dietary measures to alleviate and prevent disease. They admit themselves that perhaps the medical profession has paid too little attention to this subject in the past.

Many doctors believe that more knowledge of nutrition is needed in order to combat "food fads." For example, Dr. Robert E. Olson, of the University of Pittsburgh (who differs seriously with me on theory and dietary planning), has written that it is necessary "to improve the standards of the practice of clinical nutrition by physicians in our country." His statement was published in *Nutrition Reviews* (Vol. 16: April, 1958). He went on to say: "Unfortunately, many practitioners of medicine are not fully informed in the field of nutrition and diet therapy, and hence are not prepared to consult with patients about the faulty diet practices which constitute the basis of faddism." Dr. Olson advocates "improved teaching of nutrition in medical school and in post-graduate activities."

Research Begins in American Homes

Training more doctors to specialize in the field of nutrition is important—but tests must be conducted by the people themselves in their own homes. You and I must examine our own eating habits and give the medical scientists an honest report about our present dietary customs. Only by analyzing our present meals and menus can the expert nutritionists discover our mistakes.

A nationwide survey, a research program, is desperately needed. Let's investigate the daily diet of American families. What are the most common nutritional errors being made by the average housewife when she purchases and prepares food? Let's learn the truth, and then take corrective action!

Today there is some encouraging news to report . . . a good sign for the future. As this book goes to press, a very important research survey has been started across the nation. It will be the largest medical study ever conducted in the history of the United States.

This giant research project began in January of 1959 and will continue for several years. It will be directed by the American Cancer Society—but the statistics and information collected will also be helpful to combat heart disorders, tuberculosis and other diseases.

Some 50,000 volunteer workers will visit 500,000 homes throughout the nation! These volunteers from the American Cancer Society will be armed with questionnaires. They will ring doorbells everywhere, and they will ask direct questions about personal habits and family backgrounds.

Each family will be asked about their diet, sleeping habits, exercise, occupations, height, weight, heredity, etc. This will be a very broad survey, on many subjects that can affect a person's health. The questions will give a complete picture of the family's environment and daily way of life.

Think of it! We will then have medical statistics covering more than one million people. One million case histories, to use as a source of knowledge. For designing and organizing this tremendously valuable research program, my congratulations go to Dr. E. Cuyler Hammond of the American Cancer Society.

I wish Dr. Hammond every success in this huge task. The survey can be a major contribution to medical science.

In the months ahead, you, the reader, may be visited by a representative of the American Cancer Society making the survey. Cooperate, by all means. Answer the questions . . . and help the medical profession compile these vital statistics. We all will benefit from the results.

(Incidentally, the initial inquiries will be made in Cleveland, Baltimore, Nashville, Harrisburg and Tampa. Then the project will continue on to other cities, and the research workers may call at your home.)

My interest in this survey is especially strong because of one key fact. The American Cancer Society was wise enough to include questions about diet. And, specifically, they will ask about the liquid portion of the diet.

According to *The New York Times*, the questionnaire will ask about the following liquids: soft drinks, alcoholic beverages, tea, and coffee. The survey will seek to learn what people are drinking with their meals. Unfortunately, the temperatures of these liquids will be overlooked, as well as how and when they are taken with relation to food.

The answers—from one million Americans—will

certainly be enlightening. I venture to predict that every expert in the field of nutrition will be shocked by the drinking habits revealed.

The liquids which the public consumes <u>during</u> meals will amaze the medical profession when they see the record. Let's hope that the findings will indicate a strong need for more detailed research along the line of food in relation to liquids and further, let's hope that it may lead to acceptance of the corrective procedures I have outlined in this book.

You have a head start. You already know my theories on how liquids and solids conflict with each other during digestion. There is no need for me to say more.

As you can see, I am heartily in favor of the nation-wide study being made by the American Cancer Society. Some outstanding and dedicated men have embarked on this vast undertaking. I hesitate to suggest any changes in the questionnaire.

However, most respectfully, I do have one suggestion to make. The questionnaire already contains inquiries about soft drinks, alcoholic beverages, tea and coffee. Let's add just one item: drinking water.

Let's ask 1,000,000 American families <u>how</u> and <u>when</u> they drink water. <u>With their meals? Before?</u> <u>Or after?</u> <u>How soon after meals?</u>

To know the water-drinking habits of so many families would be valuable information for all nutritionists to study. I have already written to Dr. Hammond, urging that these questions be included in his survey.

A Forecast for the Future

When all the results of all the surveys are tabulated, I predict a major change in our nation's attitude toward nutrition. The public is already starting to accept the idea that something is missing in our present-day food supply. Millions of Americans are already trying to augment their meals by taking vitamins and special food supplements.

This growing trend toward using vitamin capsules, etc., is at least a move in the right direction. People have finally realized that they are making dietary mistakes, and they hope that swallowing pills will somehow correct nutritional deficiencies.

The use of vitamin-mineral tablets can be helpful. But choose carefully when you buy such products. Be sure that the vitamins and ingredients came from natural sources . . . read the label on the bottle or box. Suggestions on this subject were made in Chapter XIX and I'd like to repeat just once more that the health foods described in that chapter are the better way to safeguard your health.

I realize that anyone who speaks out in favor of organic foods is immediately called a "food faddist." Critics may make this charge against me. In reply, I maintain that a "food fad" is a temporary trend that is very popular one day and forgotten the next. Certainly this label does <u>not</u> apply to organic foods and supplemental natural sources of vitamins and minerals.

Millions of people have relied on health foods for many years, dietary supplements have been <u>growing</u> in acceptance. The public has shown an <u>increasing</u> interest for several decades, and a dietary program which continues for so many years cannot be called a "fad."

More and more scientists and members of the medical profession are now realizing that organic foods can be beneficial. To measure the results—the improvement in a person's health—doctors can conduct a series of blood chemistry tests.

Take two groups of patients. Have one group follow their regular diet. Give the second group a diet which features organic foods rather than highly processed foods. Following the test, compare the two groups, and there will be a dramatic difference in their health.

I recommend a blood chemistry examination. It can serve as guide on which to base future eating habits. For example, check these three items:

1. Have a blood serum cholesterol test done. If there is a high level of cholesterol, then your diet is providing your body with too much of the wrong kind of oils. You should then correct your eating habits and change to foods which come from organic sources, or you may have to learn to abstain from oil-free liquids at mealtimes.

2. Test your blood sugar level. You may have too

much sugar in your system. Again, organic foods can help restore a proper balance of carbohydrates.

3. Have a blood count made, to learn the number of red blood cells and white blood cells. If there is a deficiency of red blood cells, you need organic foods to help fight anemia. Too many white blood cells could mean malnutrition of the bodily tissues. Combat this condition, too, by adding organic foods to your daily diet.

What Are Your Chances for a Longer Life?

All of us would like to lengthen our span of life . . . to enjoy retirement, grandchildren, travel. But what can we do to guarantee ourselves good health in our later years?

Do not be deceived by glowing reports that "everyone lives longer these days." Insurance companies are releasing charts and information which supposedly prove that the average American now has a greater life expectancy. This fact is true, but the actuary tables neglect to mention one important point. It is not so important how long we live, if our final years are ruined by chronic illness and painful diseases.

Medical science has learned many ways to ward off fatal illness . . . but meanwhile older people are suffering from more and more degenerative ailments. The afflictions of "old age" are on the increase. Heart disease, arthritis, cancer, mental illness are claiming more victims than ever before.

The only answer is to start now on a nationwide research program of preventive medicine. Before a human body degenerates, let's protect it by taking preventive measures through proper nutrition.

Let us conduct a campaign among physicians and scientists, until they agree to explore the importance of nutrition as a weapon against all diseases. Each major illness may have as many as 75 variable types, or 500 subtypes. But, basically, the primary cause of disease is malnutrition of the tissues.

If the medical profession will accept this fact—and will pursue research accordingly—then we will soon see the greatest discoveries in the history of health.

Again, the key word is research. More doctors must devote their full time to research as a career. Today, there are approximately 260,000 physicians in the United States. Yet only 20,000 of them are engaged in constant research work. Millions of dollars must be provided—by the government or the public—to increase this number of medical scientists. Our nation needs at least 45,000 experts whose only activity is to study the cause and the cure of disease.

In *The New York Times* not long ago, a statement was made that we already have enough "leads" to conquer cancer and heart disease, if there were enough research money to complete the task!

A "Manhattan Project" to Win Another War

Our nation marshaled together billions of dollars and the most intelligent scientists on earth in order to win World War II. We all can recall the famous Manhattan Project, where research produced the atom bomb. Now the time has come to create another "Manhattan Project" to fight man's battle for better health.

Every available resource in our country today should be combined in a concentrated effort, so that scientific teamwork can defeat disease.

We need a coordinated program—where all research information is pooled together—so that doctors can share their discoveries and immediately test each new method of cure.

This plan to establish a "Manhattan Project" in the field of health is not just a dream. It can be done. In fact, the groundwork has already been started. A committee has been formed in New York City to create a medical research organization of gigantic size.

Leading this campaign is Mrs. Albert D. Lasker, chairman of the National Health Education Committee, with offices in the Chrysler Building. She and her associates are raising millions of dollars to support this project. They are contacting private industry, the federal government and every possible source of funds to help in this fight.

Mrs. Lasker believes that we have enough leads to

conquer disease and that the main problem is merely to raise enough money for testing and research. Her views were explained in *The New York Times* article mentioned above. Her organization will lead a combined attack in five areas of health.

The most prevalent illnesses that kill and cripple can be classified in five categories. 1. Heart disease and arteriosclerosis (hardening of the arteries). 2. Cancer. 3. Mental illness. 4. Arthritis and metabolic diseases. 5. Neurological and blinding eye diseases.

If we can find the answers to defeat these five, then all mankind will enjoy a fabulous future. This is the goal which Mrs. Lasker and her committee have set out to achieve. The National Health Education Committee deserves our thanks for their action to meet this tremendous challenge.

As we look ahead—and see the future course of medical research—the prospects are brighter than they have been in many years. Because of the surveys described in this chapter, it appears that our nation is finally ready to wage a war against chronic illness. Millions of dollars will be spent by our federal government, through the Health, Education and Welfare Department and the National Institute of Public Health. Scientists will now receive the recognition and the financial support they need to do the job right.

And I am most optimistic that the "right" approach will include research on nutrition. I firmly believe that hospitals, clinics and research centers will turn more and more toward dietary methods—will discover that a wide range of diseases can be conquered by nutritional measures.

While this progress is certain to occur, it may take a few more years for the theory to be accepted. You and I can't wait even that long. We must start now, today, to correct our dietary mistakes. We can practice good nutrition immediately. We already know how.

Until the time when the statements in this book become acknowledged by scientists everywhere, you have a head start. You can enjoy better health from the moment you adopt the dietary procedures that have been outlined here. Your key to a new way of life is the ten-point program shown in Chapter I. Study it . . . act on it.

Examine yourself, using the checklist of symptoms found in Chapter 2. When you know the state of your present health, follow the plan of diet and notice the improvement.

Protect yourself and protect your family by understanding how to eat and drink. Learn how to use correct diet as preventive medicine and how to use common sense for better health.

Now you are on your own. This book has given you the knowledge, the opportunity for self-help. Just consider the facts, and your decision will be easy to make. Choose a happier, healthier life . . . the common sense way!

SEND A COPY OF THIS BOOK TO A FRIEND

Somewhere amongst your many friends and relatives you may know a person or two who is interested in diet and good health. Someone who would appreciate receiving a copy of this book GOOD HEALTH & COMMON SENSE. It is a nice gesture . . . giving additional, and maybe helpful, information to a person already interested in this subject. And maybe it would be a good gift for someone who could use it . . . but doesn't realize it yet.

For additional copies we suggest you first try your local bookstores or department stores. But if they happen to be out of stock we will be pleased to receive your orders directly, and they will be shipped immediately, postpaid. The price is $8.95 plus .50¢ postage and handling. Just drop a letter with your address, or the address of the person you want to receive the book, to us.

THE WITKOWER PRESS, INC.
Box 2296, Bishops Corner
West Hartford, Conn. 06117